Oklahoma Notes

Basic-Sciences Review for Medical Licensure
Developed at
The University of Oklahoma, College of Medicine

Suitable Reviews for:
National Board of Medical Examiners (NBME), Part I
Medical Sciences Knowledge Profile (MSKP)
Foreign Medical Graduate Examination in the Medical Sciences (FMGEMS)

Oklahoma Notes

Pharmacology

Edited by
Joanne I. Moore

With Contributions by
John M. Carney   H. Dix Christensen
K. Roger Hornbrook   Michael C. Koss   Charles F. Meier, Jr.
Joanne I. Moore   Lester A. Reinke   Lora E. Rikans

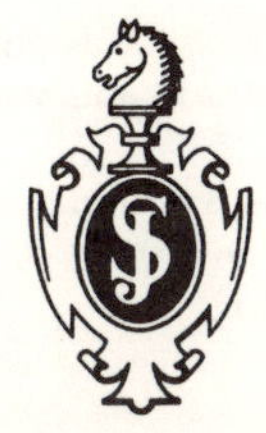

Springer-Verlag
New York Berlin Heidelberg
London Paris Tokyo

Joanne I. Moore, Ph.D.
Department of Pharmacology
College of Medicine
Health Sciences Center
The University of Oklahoma
Oklahoma City, OK 73190
USA

Library of Congress Cataloging in Publication Data
Pharmacology.
  (Oklahoma notes)
  1. Pharmacology—Examinations, questions, etc.
I. Moore, Joanne I. II. Carney, John M. III. Series.
[DNLM: 1. Pharmacology. 2. Pharmacology—examination
questions. QV 4 P53605]
RM105.P473   1986   615'.1   86-22074

Printed in the United States of America.

9 8 7 6 5 4 (Corrected fourth printing, 1988)

ISBN 0-387-96332-4 Springer-Verlag New York Berlin Heidelberg
ISBN 3-540-96332-4 Springer-Verlag Berlin Heidelberg New York

Preface to the
Oklahoma Notes

In 1973, the University of Oklahoma College of Medicine instituted a requirement for passage of the Part I National Boards for promotion to the third year. To assist students in preparation for this examination, a two-week review of the basic sciences was added to the curriculum in 1975. Ten review texts were written by the faculty: four in anatomical sciences and one each in the other six basic sciences. Self-instructional quizzes were also developed by each discipline and administered during the review period.

The first year the course was instituted the Total Score performance on National Boards Part I increased 60 points, with the relative standing of the school changing from 56th to 9th in the nation. The performance of the class has remained near the national candidate mean (500) since then, with a mean over the 12 years of 502 and a range of 467 to 537. This improvement in our own students' performance has been documented (Hyde et al: Performance on NBME Part I examination in relation to policies regarding use of test. J. Med. Educ. 60:439–443, 1985).

A questionnaire was administered to one of the classes after they had completed the boards; 82% rated the review books as the most beneficial part of the course. These texts have been recently updated and rewritten and are now available for use by all students of medicine who are preparing for comprehensive examinations in the Basic Medical Sciences.

RICHARD M. HYDE, Ph.D.
Executive Editor

<u>PREFACE</u>

More than ten years ago, the faculty members of the Department of Pharmacology at the University of Oklahoma College of Medicine developed a review book of medical pharmacology in response to requests from our second year medical students who were preparing to sit for the Part I examination of the National Board of Medical Examiners. The students expressed a need for an organized approach to cope with the volume of basic science curricular material presented during the first two years. Therefore, our review book was not designed to provide a comprehensive text on pharmacology, but rather to provide the students with a significant core of information, as a refresher, after they had successfully completed a basic course in pharmacology.

This book represents a major revision of our review of medical pharmacology. The book has been reorganized, updated and expanded to provide current information on major new drugs and information on older drug groups that typically are covered on licensure examinations. The book also has been expanded to include a large number of new questions for self-examination. The faculty have endeavored to retain a reasonably concise, relevant and readable review book that will provide the students with a thorough review of pharmacology. Students are advised to refer to comprehensive textbooks, as needed, to fill in any gaps in their knowledge which may be disclosed by the self-examinations.

We wish to acknowledge the help of several contributors to the original version of the review book. These include former members of the faculty, Daniel M. Byrd, III, Ph.D., Andrew T. Chiu, Ph.D. and Walter N. Piper, Ph.D., as well as a Visiting Professor from The University of Michigan, Henry H. Swain, M.D.

We wish to offer our special thanks to Annie M. Harjo for her skills with the word processor and for remaining calm and unflappable during our efforts in assembling this book.

Joanne I. Moore, Ph.D.

<u>SECTION VII</u>:   <u>CHEMOTHERAPY</u> (J.I. Moore, L.A. Reinke and L.E. Rikans)

<u>SECTION VIII</u>:   <u>MISCELLANEOUS DRUGS</u> (J.I. Moore, L.A. Reinke and L.E. Rikans)

SECTION I: <u>GENERAL PRINCIPLES</u>

I. <u>Mechanisms of Drug Action</u>

    A. Known physical or chemical interactions

        1. Osmotic cathartics and osmotic diuretics

        2. Antacids

    B. Unknown mechanism related to a physical property of the agent, <u>i.e.</u>, oil: H_2O solubility which determines cellular concentration.

        1. Most general anesthetics agents

    C. Molecular site of interaction——drug receptor

        1. Drugs usually not accumulated at site of action.

        2. Drugs usually do not directly affect known enzymatic pathways or structural elements within cells, although important exceptions occur in chemotherapy and some metabolic effects of drugs.

        3. Most drug effects are produced by interaction with a cellular binding site of generally unknown chemical composition. By the translation of binding into an observable effect the site is a drug receptor, by definition.

            a. binding not translated into an effect is a storage site, <u>i.e.</u>, plasma protein.

            b. binding at both receptors and storage sites is usually reversible and occurs by low energy forces. A few examples of covalent binding are known: organophosphorus cholinesterase inhibitors and some chemotherapeutic agents.

                1. covalent binding of drugs to cellular constituents may result in toxicity <u>(i.e.,</u> cellular necrosis, allergic potential, carcinogenesis).

            c. the receptor normally interacts with endogenous substances <u>(i.e.,</u> neurotransmitters, hormones, autacoids, peptides, etc.); thus the binding of drugs to the receptor requires structural specificity and often stereospecificity.

            d. selective effect of a drug for an organ system is related to the presence of a specific receptor; the type of response is related to the organ's normal function.

            e. characterization of receptors

                1. mobile receptors - steroid hormones

a. complex formed in cytoplasm and derivative goes to nucleus.

b. production of effect related to synthesis of a specific m-RNA and of new protein molecules.

c. transduction involves interaction of receptor with DNA; amplification involves the number of new protein molecules synthesized.

2. fixed receptors - catecholamines, acetylcholine and other endogenous substances, or drugs.

a. interaction generally occurs in plasma membrane, but thyroxin has a receptor fixed in nucleus.

b. transduction and amplification: second messengers

1. cyclic nucleotides and protein phosphorylation

a. guanine nucleotide binding protein (G-protein; N-factor) is carrier of information from membrane to adenylate cyclase; cyclic-AMP carries information to protein kinases in cytoplasm. G-protein also transfers information at sites other than adenylate cyclase.

b. action of cyclic-GMP not defined well, but involves protein phosphorylation.

c. non-cyclic nucleotide dependent protein kinases (kinase-C and tyrosine kinase).

2. calcium ion

a. membrane gating affected by fluidity or phosphoinositol turnover.

b. calmodulin as effector; increased protein phosphorylation or phosphodiesterase activation.

c. voltage-dependent and other calcium channels.

3. low molecular weight peptides formed in membrane (_i.e._, after insulin reacts with receptor).

4. prostaglandins and related compounds; free radicals.

c. desensitization: tolerance; tachyphalaxis

1. slow regeneration from inactive receptor form.

2. formation of endogenous inhibitor.

3. negative co-operativity of drug-receptor binding.

4. agonist-mediated decrease in receptor number: down regulation, internalization.

5. depletion of "second" messenger or endogenously released factor.

6. desensitization does not occur with antagonists.

d. pathologic states of receptor function

1. immunological decrease in number; myasthenia gravis, asthma.

2. agonist-mediated decrease in number; diabetes mellitus.

3. loss of coupling factor (G-protein) between membrane and cytosol; pseudohypoparathyroidism.

e. classification of drug-receptor interations

1. agonist - drugs producing a response by binding to a receptive site. The ability to "stimulate" this site is a property called efficacy or intrinsic activity, and is independent of affinity. Generally have structural similarity to endogenous compounds.

2. antagonist - drugs that act by inhibiting the action of known endogenous mediators. These are agents with high affinity for the receptor but produce no effect because they lack efficacy. Some drugs classified as agonists may in fact block unknown endogenous substances. Best known antagonists are those which interact with the autonomic nervous system. Structural similarity to agonists may not be apparent because antagonism results from hydrophobic interactions with the receptor.

3. partial agonists - drugs with less efficacy than agonists, and thus, produce a smaller maximal response; can also be considered partial antagonists (mixed agonist-antagonist). The recognition of efficacy or intrinsic activity may be a property of the coupling factor and not the receptor.

f. quantitation of drug-receptor interactions

1. usually done with dose-response curves in which log dose is plotted against response; conceptually, the kinetics are the same as enzyme kinetics because the mass action principle is involved in both cases.

2. this plot gives sigmoid curves which are linear through middle 66% of curve.

3. most accurate point is the dose producing a 50%
   response (ED_{50}) and comparisons between drugs made
   at this point. With full agonists, observed ED_{50}
   may be considerably less than dissociation constant
   due to "spare" receptors; i.e., full response with
   less than 100% occupation.

4. Figure 1 shows, dose-response curves plotted
   logarithmically to two agonists with different
   potencies.

Figure 1

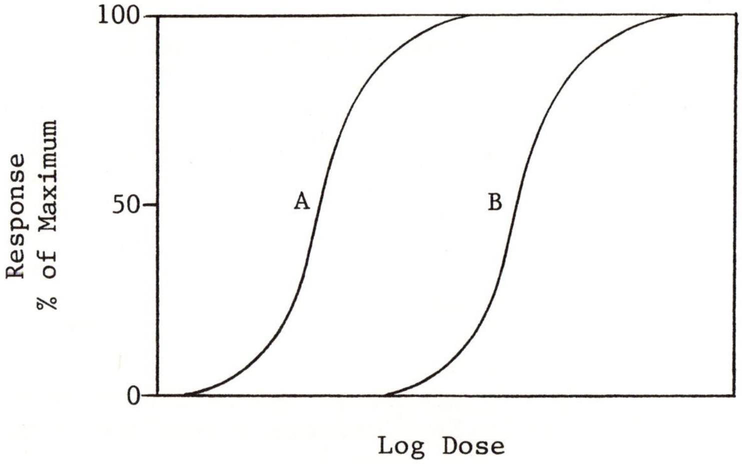

5. potency of agonists related to apparent affinity of
   drug for receptor; a more potent drug is not
   necessarily a better drug.

6. antagonists can bind to a receptor site or a site
   near the receptor and thus limit its interaction
   with agonists.

   a. competitive antagonists shift the dose-response
      curve for agonists to the right but do not
      decrease the maximal response obtainable. In
      figure 2, curve S is the response to agonist R
      in the presence of a competitive antagonist.

Figure 2

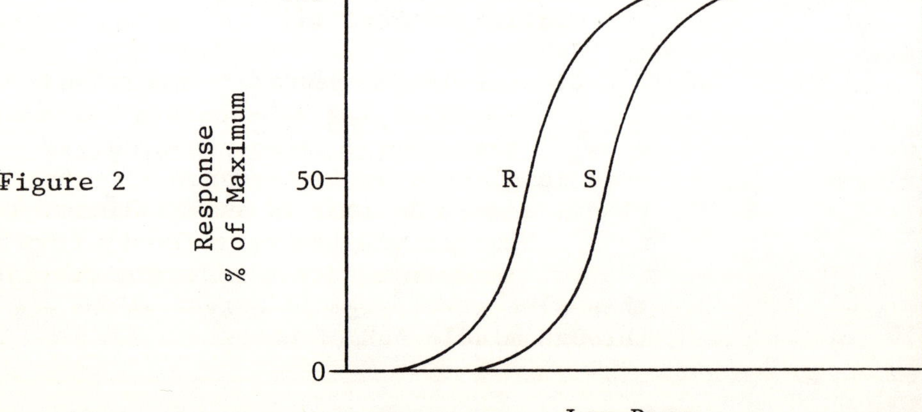

b. non-competitive antagonists act at a site near the receptor to alter its configuration and both shift the curve to the right and decrease the maximal response obtainable. In figure 3, curve Y is the response to agonist X in the presence of a non-competitive antagonist.

Figure 3

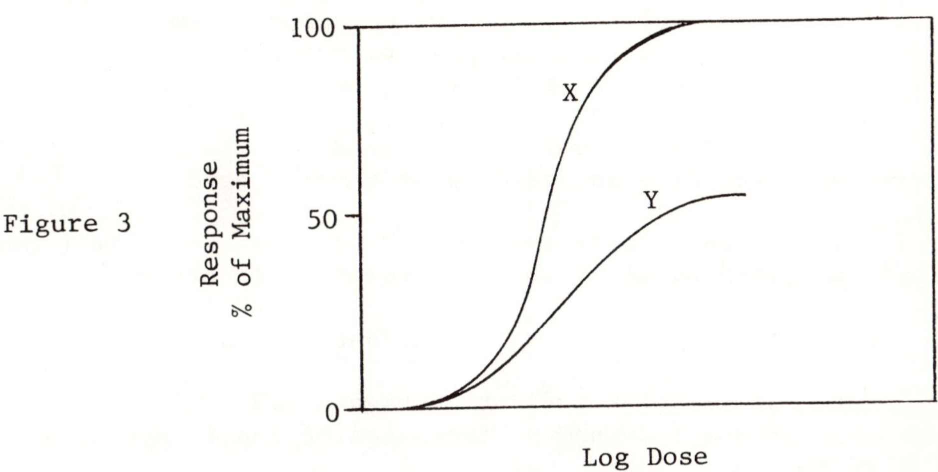

c. competitive-irreversible antagonists combine covalently with the receptor site and also shift the curve to the right and decrease the maximal response obtainable. The dose-response would be the same as figure 3. Also, figure 3 could depict dose-response curves for a partial agonist-Y, and full agonist-X.

d. antagonism of a drug effect by another agent can occur at sites other than the receptor through chemical interactions or opposing functional processes.

7. therapeutic index

a. an initial evaluation of the safety of drugs in lower animals.

b. ratio of LD_{50}:ED_{50}: might also use toxic effect rather than lethal.

1. curves for toxicity and effect must be parallel for an accurate estimation of the therapeutic index.

2. not all toxic effects observed subsequently in man will be detected by this screening procedure, i.e., allergic reactions.

II. <u>Absorption</u>

    A. From gastro-intestinal tract

        1. Amount absorbed depends on:

            a. physical state and solubility in enteral fluids.
            b. pKa of drug.
            c. lipid solubility of the unionized form.
            d. destruction of drug by gut constituents.
            e. blood flow in gut wall.
            f. transit time.
            g. binding to food.
            h. precipitation of drug by gastric acid.

        2. In general, acids absorbed better than bases in stomach; bases absorbed better than acids in small intestine.

        3. Absorption of both acids and bases occur in small intestine because:

            a. pH is not inordinately high – 5.3.
            b. blood flow and surface area of small intestine are large.

        4. Bases can be accumulated in the stomach from plasma by ion-trapping. Unionized drug diffuses across wall, ionizes at low pH and cannot diffuse back; the converse occurs for acids.

        5. Some drugs are ineffective after oral administration because splanchnic blood flow passes through the liver and metabolism occurs (first-pass effect).

    B. After injection

        1. Absorption said to be faster after i.m. than after s.c.

            a. blood flow greater.

            b. surface area greater.

        2. To decrease rate of absorption.

            a. give drug as an insoluble salt or in oil i.m., or s.c., implantation of compressed pellets s.c.

            b. decrease blood flow by vasoconstriction.

        3. Give highly irritating or tissue-toxic drugs i.v.; all drugs given i.v. should be injected slowly.

    C. Other routes

        1. Skin – mostly of toxicological importance or for local effect except for administration of scopolamine, nitroglycerin, and clonidine.

        2. Lungs – gaseous anesthetics and aerosols (local action).

III. <u>Distribution of Drugs</u>

    A. Volume of distribution

        1. $V.D. = \dfrac{\text{dose (mg)}}{\text{plasma concentration (mg/L)}}$

        2. This calculation gives V.D. in Liters for a one compartment model.

        3. Dividing also by body weight gives value in percent of body weight.

        4. Calculated volume may or may not correspond to a body water space.

        5. Binding of a drug to a storage site can give a value greater than total body water.

        6. V.D. contributes to the rate of elimination of a drug in that the larger the V.D., the slower the rate of elimination.

    B. Importance of unequal distribution

        1. Initial distribution to organs which receive a large fraction of cardiac output; subsequent redistribution to less well perfused organs may terminate effect (i.e. thiopental).

        2. Blood brain barrier: small capillary pores and glial cells keep compounds with low lipid solubility from interstitial space of brain.

        3. Drug storage sites

           a. tissue fat, protein, nucleic acids.

           b. plasma protein.

               1. drugs are primarily bound to albumin, but basic drugs also bind to <u>alpha</u>-acid glycoprotein.

               2. drug bound to protein is inactive but can serve as storage site and prolong the effect; however, if drug eliminated by active process, the effect is shortened.

               3. less binding and more free drug may occur with hypoalbuminemia or uremia.

               4. drug interactions may result because of displacement of a drug bound to plasma protein by another drug if:

                   a. bound drug has a low therapeutic index.
                   b. bound drug has a small volume of distribution.
                   c. if more than 95% of the drug in plasma is protein bound.

IV. <u>Excretion of Drugs</u>

    A. Most important route is the kidney.

1. Drugs filtered at glomerulus are variably reabsorbed from tubules depending on:

   a. pH of urine and pKa of drug.

   b. lipid solubility.

   c. clearance can vary between zero and GFR (130 ml/min).

2. Highly ionized acids and bases are actively secreted by tubular cells and clearance can approach renal plasma flow (600 ml/min).

3. Neonates and elderly have low GFR and renal blood flow.

B. Enterohepatic cycle

   1. Active secretion of a conjugated drug into the bile, _i.e._, glucuronic acid derivative of a phenol.

   2. Unconjugated drug liberated in small intestine by hydrolysis and free drug reabsorbed into plasma.

   3. Some drug escapes reabsorption and appears in feces.

C. Lungs – primarily anesthetic agents

   1. Blood/air partition coefficient.

      a. large value – slow excretion. Rate of pulmonary circulation limiting.

      b. small value – more rapid excretion. Rate of pulmonary ventilation limiting.

D. Skin – through sweat glands and may result in direct irritation or allergic reactions

V. <u>Determinants of plasma concentration and dosage schedules</u>

   A. Rates of elimination

      1. Most drugs disappear from plasma by processes (<u>i.e.</u> metabolism, secretion, filtration) which are concentration dependent (first order kinetics).

a. plot of log plasma concentration against time is a straight line (figure 4).

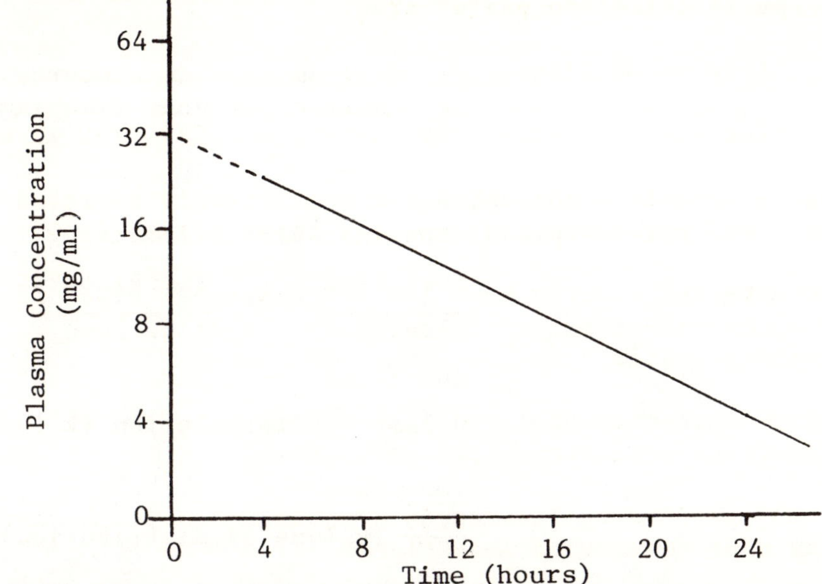

Figure 4

b. constant percentage of the drug lost per unit time as long as no elimination route is saturated; this value equivalent to the elimination rate constant (k_e).

c. the biologic half-life is constant at all non-saturating plasma concentrations, and is related to ke:

$$t\tfrac{1}{2} = \frac{0.69}{k_e}$$

d. k_e related to clearance of drug from plasma and volume of distribution:

$$k_e = \frac{\text{clearance (ml/min)}}{\text{volume of distribution (ml)}} = \frac{1}{\text{min}} \quad \text{or percentage of drug lost per unit time}$$

e. these considerations apply only to free drug in plasma and not that bound to plasma protein.

2. Drugs which saturate routes of elimination will disappear from plasma in a non-concentration dependent manner (zero order kinetics).

a. plot of log plasma concentration against time may appear linear, particularly at early time periods, but it is illusory. Check graphs closely.

b. constant amount of drug lost per unit time; there is not an equivalent elimination rate constant.

c. the biologic half-life is not constant but depends on the concentration; the higher the concentration, the longer the half-life (dose-dependent kinetics).

d. drugs in this category will have first order kinetics whenever the elimination process is no longer saturated.

3. Accumulation of drugs in body

a. drugs will accumulate until amount administered per unit time is equal to the amount eliminated per unit time (amount in = amount out)

b. amount in = dose/time
amount out = plasma concentration (clearance)

$$\text{Plasma concentration} = \frac{\text{dose/time}}{\text{clearance}} \quad \text{or} \quad \frac{\text{infusion rate}}{\text{clearance}}$$

$$= \frac{\text{dose/time}}{\text{volume of distribution } (k_e)}$$

$$= \frac{\text{dose/time}}{\frac{0.69}{t\frac{1}{2}}} \text{ (volume of distribution)}$$

$$= \frac{1.5 \, (t\frac{1}{2}) \, (\text{dose/time})}{\text{volume of distribution}}$$

c. this value is the average plasma concentration; the fluctuation around this concentration is equal to the dose corrected for volume of distribution.

d. the time to reach steady-state concentration is related to $t\frac{1}{2}$; 90% of steady state in 3.3 half-lives, 94% in 4 half-lives and 99% in 6-8 half-lives. Drugs with long half-lives (days) may require priming doses to avoid delay in therapeutic effect.

e. to change concentration, it is generally better to increase frequency of dosing rather than amount to avoid toxic effects.

f. drug eliminated rapidly ($t\frac{1}{2}$ = 4 hr or less) usually given by i.v. infusion or by slowly absorbed preparation.

g. no simple prediction of plasma concentration can be made for drugs eliminated by zero order kinetics. Toxic concentrations can accumulate more quickly and be lost more slowly than drugs which follow first order kinetics.

h. drug dosage in renal disease

1. applies to drugs excreted primarily (more than 50%) unchanged by kidney and not those eliminated by other processes.

2. initial dose same as normal patient.

3. either dose decreased or dose interval increased in proportion to decrease in renal clearance of creatinine and percentage of drug eliminated unchanged by kidney.

i. no basis for correction of dosage schedules related to hepatic disease.

VI. <u>Metabolism of Drugs</u>

A. Sites of metabolism

1. Quantitatively the most important site is the endoplasmic reticulum (microsomes) of the liver but metabolism also occurs in other organelles, such as mitochondria (MAO), probably lysosomes, and in the cytosol (alcohol dehydrogenase and diamine oxidase).

2. All tissues have the ability to metabolize some foreign compounds by oxidation and/or conjugation; after liver, the most active sites of drug metabolism are kidney, lung and intestine.

B. Types of reactions can be classified as non-synthetic (phase I) and synthetic (phase II or conjugation reactions).

1. Non-synthetic reactions:

a. oxidations, reductions and hydrolysis.

b. most oxidations and reductions are catalyzed by the mixed-function oxidase enzymes in the endoplasmic reticulum and are characterized by requirements for NADPH and molecular oxygen, and the involvement of cytochromes P-450, NADPH-cytochrome P-450 reductase and phospholipid.

c. these reactions generally make a compound more water soluble and more readily excreted but not necessarily less active. The metabolic product may be more active or possess new toxic properties. Many potentially carcinogenic compounds are activated by this enzymatic mechanism.

d. compounds produced by these reactions may be excreted as such or processed further by conjugation, thus the term phase II metabolism. After conjugation, the drugs are usually pharmacologically inactive and not metabolized further because they are too water soluble to penetrate to sites of metabolism. Some carcinogens may be active in conjugated form.

2. Synthetic reactions

a. these reactions include conjugation with glucuronic acid (occurs in endoplasmic reticulum), amino acids (glycine, glutamine), sulfate, methylation, acetylation or glutathione (mercapturic acids).

b. in most cases, the conjugating group is activated, i.e., UDP-glucuronic acid and acetyl-CoA; but for the conjugation of organic acids with amino acids, the organic acid is converted to a coenzyme A derivative.

C. Factors influencing drug metabolism

1. Age - fetuses, newborns, and the elderly do not metabolize drugs as well as adults.

2. Species - generalization from lower animals to man may not be valid.

3. Genetic background variations in metabolism of succinylcholine, isoniazid and phenytoin can result in toxicity with usual doses of the drugs.

4. Disease states

   a. cirrhosis can decrease metabolism.

   b. porphyria - some drugs increase the activity of ALA synthase.

5. Inhibitors of drug metabolism

   a. may lead to accumulation of concomitantly administered drugs.

   b. competitive inhibition between drug substrate for the microsomal enzymes is readily demonstrated _in vitro_ and probably occurs _in vivo_.

   c. clinically significant interactions due to decreased metabolism have been reported for anticoagulants, phenytoin and oral hypoglycemic agents, which interact with a diverse group of drugs. These compounds probably get singled out because they are taken chronically in amounts sufficient to saturate drug-metabolizing enzymes and have a low therapeutic index; rather small changes in the plasma concentration may lead to a severe, recognizable toxic reaction.

6. Inducers of drug metabolism

   a. a wide variety of compounds increase the activity of the hepatic microsomal drug metabolizing system. The result is a decrease in pharmacological activity of other concomitantly administered drugs.

   b. both phase I and phase II reactions may be induced.

   c. magnitude of induction depends on basal level of activity; a two-fold change is common in patients.

   d. return to normal activity takes several days to several weeks.

7. Hormones - may induce drug metabolism, and are physiological substrates of mixed-function oxidases

   a. sex steroids.

      b.   corticosteroids.

    8. Nutritional factors – may alter Phase I or Phase II reactions due to the presence of inducing agents in the diet or by affecting the availability of precursors for biosynthesis of cofactors (e.g., carbohydrates for the biosynthesis of UDP-glucuronic acid).

D. Specific drug biotransformation reactions

    1. Oxidation (Phase I)

        a.   aromatic hydroxylation.
        b.   N-dealkylation.
        c.   O-dealkylation.
        d.   desulfuration.
        e.   alkyl oxidation.
        f.   oxidative deamination.
        g.   sulfoxidation.
        h.   epoxidation.

    2. Reduction (Phase I) – may be catalyzed primarily in the gut by anaerobic bacteria

        a.   azo- and nitro-compounds.
        b.   organic nitrates.

    3. Hydrolysis (Phase I)

        a.   esterases.
        b.   amidases.
        c.   occurs in plasma, liver cytosol, as well as in other tissues.

    4. Conjugation (Phase II)

        a.   glucuronidation.
        b.   glycine conjugation.
        c.   glutathione conjugation.
        d.   mercapturic acid conjugation (breakdown product of glutathione conjugation).
        e.   acetylation.
        f.   sulfation.
        g.   methylation.
        h.   glutamine conjugation.

VII. <u>Pharmacogenetics</u>

A. Genes and Drug Metabolism

    1. Prolonged apnea with succinylcholine; atypical plasma cholinesterase; autosomal recessive, 1 in 2500.

    2. Rapid or slow acetylation (isoniazid, hydralazine, sulfamethazine, etc.); liver N-acetyl transferase; slow acetylation is autosomal recessive, 1 in 2; lupoid reactions from hydralazine and procainamide are more common in slow acetylators.

3. Abnormal metabolism by the hepatic microsomal enzyme system; toxicity results from accumulation of parent drug or production of an alternate (more toxic) metabolite; phenytoin, phenacetin, dicumarol, tolbutamide.

B. Genes and Target Tissues

1. Drug-induced red cell hemolysis; many drugs involved, primaquine is classic example; hemolytic drug reactions are related to glucose-6-phosphate dehydrogenase deficiency, methemoglobin reductase deficiency or abnormal hemoglobins; 100 million people carry the trait, 100 variants are known (all sex-linked).

2. Malignant hyperthermia; cause unknown; muscular rigidity, tachycardia, marked hyperthermia, often fatal; halothane, inhalation anesthetics, succinylcholine have been implicated; autosomal dominant, 1 in 20,000.

3. Warfarin resistance; diminished affinity of receptor for warfarin and increased affinity for vitamin K, autosomal dominant, extremely rare.

REVIEW QUESTIONS

ONE BEST ANSWER

Drugs A and B have the following dose-response curves. Answer the
following questions considering each question independently.

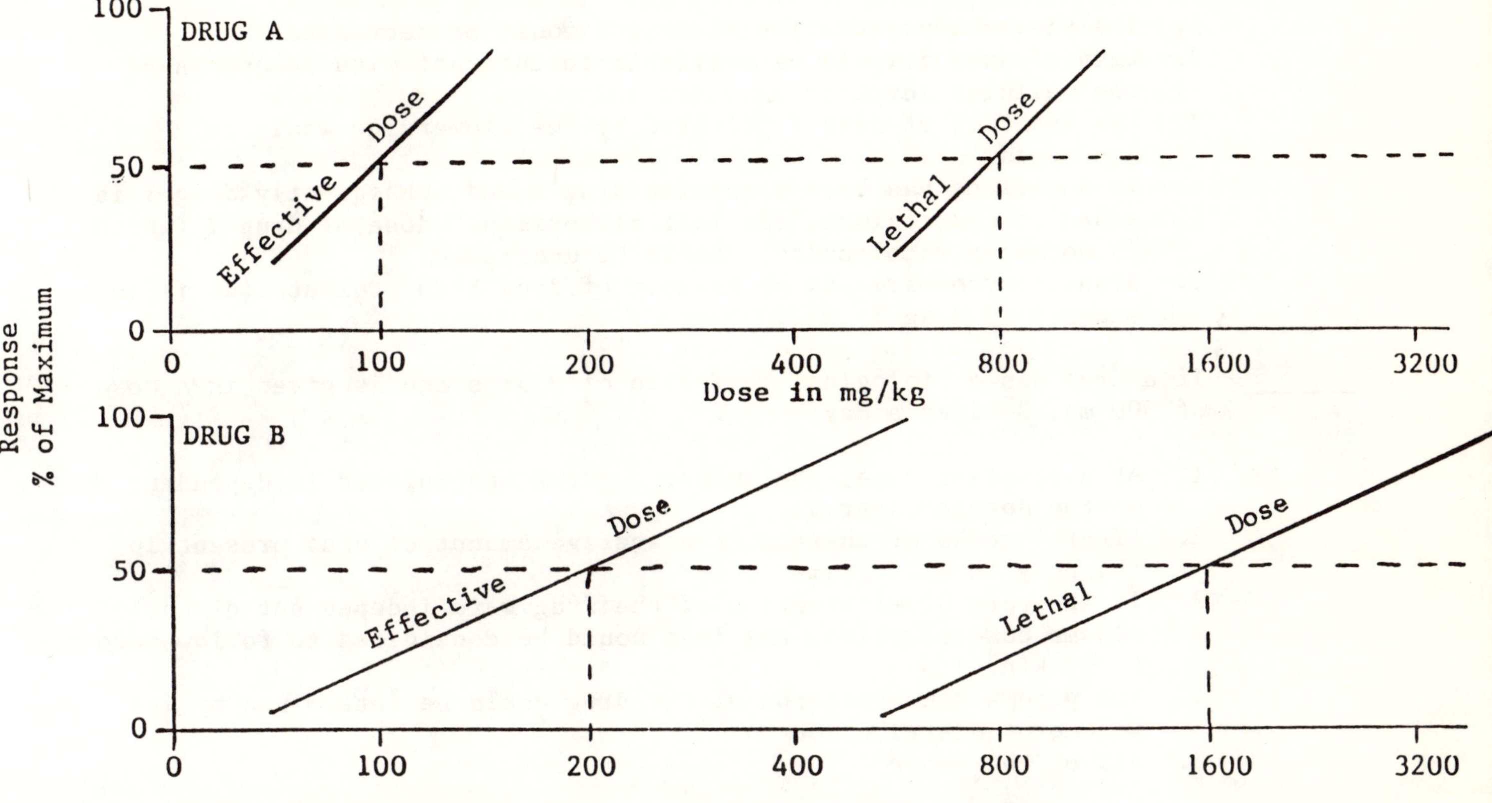

1. _______ Which drug has the larger "therapeutic index"?

    1. Drug A
    2. Drug B
    3. Drug A and drug B are equal
    4. Indeterminant

2. _______ Which drug has the larger potential safety factor in clinical use?

    1. Drug A
    2. Drug B
    3. Drug A and drug B are equal
    4. Indeterminant

3. _______ Which drug is the most potent?

    1. Drug A
    2. Drug B
    3. Drug A and drug B are equal
    4. Indeterminant

<u>ONE BEST ANSWER</u>

4. _______ Drug interactions generally fall into the category of altered absorption, distribution, metabolism or excretion of one drug as influenced by another. If drug X displaces drug Y from serum albumin (because they share the same binding sites and albumin has a greater affinity for drug X) all of the following statements are true EXCEPT?

1. The plasma concentration of drug Y would be decreased
2. Less of drug Y would be available to interact with receptors at the cellular level
3. The quantity of drug Y filtered by the glomerulus would be increased
4. If a patient has been receiving drug X and subsequently drug Y is added to the regimen, the initial "priming" dose of drug Y (which is normally recommended) should be decreased.
5. Bishydroxycoumarin is an example of drug X and tolbutamide is an example of drug Y

5. _______ If a drug has a biological half-life of 3 days and is given in a dose of 500 mg, 3 times a day:

1. At a constant dose, the amount of drug accumulated is dependent on the dosage interval
2. After 4 weeks of therapy, the average amount of drug present in the body is 6.75 grams
3. If the rate of elimination of the drug were independent of the plasma concentration, the loss would be considered to follow zero order kinetics
4. The plasma concentration of the drug would be determined by its volume of distribution
5. All of the above

6. _______ Oxidation of drugs in the hepatic endoplasmic reticulum depends upon:

1. S-adenosyl methionine
2. Uridinediphosphate glucuronic acid
3. Acetyl coenzyme A
4. Hepatic cholinesterase
5. None of the above

7. _______ Which <u>one</u> of the following would be <u>most</u> important in determining the amount of drug present in the brain?

1. Whether or not the drug increases cardiac output
2. Lipoid solubility of the drug
3. The amount of drug bound to plasma protein
4. The rate at which the drug is metabolized or eliminated

<u>ONE BEST ANSWER</u>

8. _______ Metabolism of a drug by the microsomal oxidation system in the liver:

1. Always results in a more polar metabolite
2. Requires the presence of NADPH and molecular oxygen
3. Can be increased by the concomitant administration of many drugs, such as phenobarbital
4. May be deficient in the new-born infant
5. All of the above

9. _______ All of the following statements are correct descriptions of drug conjugation mechanisms EXCEPT:

1. Either the drug or the endogenous substance with which it is conjugated must be activated prior to conjugation
2. Conjugation is usually followed by oxidation of the drug
3. The product of conjugation is usually a strongly ionized acid, readily excreted
4. Some conjugation mechanisms are not fully active at birth

10. _______ In man, the most common route of metabolism of drugs bearing an organic acid (-COOH) group is:

1. Acetylation
2. Ester hydrolysis
3. Sulfate conjugation
4. Amino acid conjugation
5. Oxidative decarboxylation

11. _______ In patients homozygous for the plasma cholinesterase variant called "atypical":

1. The action of an ordinary dose of succinylcholine lasts for a couple of minutes instead of about an hour
2. The rate of hydrolysis of succinylcholine is much greater than normal
3. The affinity between succinylcholine and the esterase is much less than normal
4. Ordinary doses of succinylcholine have very little effect
5. Acetylation of procainamide is slow

<u>**ONE BEST ANSWER**</u>

A new antiarrhythmic agent, "Rhythmstat," is given i.v. to a patient in a dose of 500 mg. The EKG is monitored and blood samples taken for analysis of plasma concentrations. The following concentrations were reported from the laboratory; concentration of free drug in μg/ml.

Time after <u>administration</u>-hours:

0.5	1	2	3	4	5	6	7	8
4.5	4.0	3.4	2.8	2.4	2.0	1.7	1.4	1.3

The EKG tracing showed changes in myocardial conduction for 30 minutes after administration which were indicative of the toxic effect of "Rhythmstat". The patient's PVC's were not apparent in the EKG until 5 hours after the drug was given i.v. The information from the drug company contains no data on the metabolism or renal clearance of the drug. The patient has no pre-existing liver or kidney disease.

12. _______ The apparent volume of distribution of "Rhythmstat" is about:

1. 40 liters
2. 100 liters
3. 200 liters
4. 400 liters

13. _______ If the clearance of "Rhythmstat" were only by the kidney, the value calculated would suggest that:

1. It was filtered and completely reabsorbed
2. It was filtered and incompletely reabsorbed
3. It was filtered and not reabsorbed
4. It was filtered and actively secreted, and thus could be used to measure renal plasma flow
5. It was filtered and actively secreted but could not be used to measure renal plasma flow

14. _______ The resident starts an i.v. infusion at a rate of 1.5 mg/min. The EKG is monitored every 30 minutes. When would the drug accumulate to a concentration sufficient to see the first signs of toxicity?

1. A toxic concentration is not reached at this rate of infusion
2. 4-5 hrs
3. 7-8 hrs
4. 13-14 hrs
5. 29-30 hrs

<u>ONE BEST ANSWER</u>

15. ________ The patient is sent home with an oral preparation of the drug. You
have decided to maintain the average plasma concentration half-way
between the toxic and minimal therapeutic plasma concentrations, and
to give the drug every eight hours. The dose the patient would take
would be within 50 mg of:

    1. 100 mg
    2. 200 mg
    3. 400 mg
    4. 800 mg
    5. 1 gram

16. ________ If the dose of "Rhythmstat" were changed to 100 mg i.v. every hour,
in the steady-state situation the fluctuation in plasma concentration
each hour would be about:

    1. 0.1 µg/ml
    2. 1 µg/ml
    3. 10 µg/ml
    4. 100 µg/ml
    5. 1000 µg/ml

17. ________ If the product information for a drug states that the drug is
oxidized by hepatic microsomal enzymes, it is referring to reactions
occurring in:

    1. The inner mitochondrial membrane
    2. The membranes of the nuclear envelope
    3. The membranes of the endoplasmic reticulum
    4. A spherical membrane-bound organelle closely associated with
       peroxisomes
    5. Soluble cytoplasmic enzymes

18. ________ All of the following statements are true of competitive irreversible
antagonists EXCEPT:

    1. Concomitant incubation of the organ with the competitive
       irreversible antagonist and a high (100 times the ED_{50})
       concentration of the agonist will substantially prevent binding
       of the antagonist
    2. They decrease the maximal response to the agonist
    3. They have affinity for the receptor, but no intrinsic activity
    4. The change in the shape of the dose-response curve is consistent
       with an increase in total number of receptors

<u>MULTIPLE TRUE–FALSE</u>
Directions: For each of the statements below, <u>ONE</u> or <u>MORE</u> of the completions
given is correct.

    1 – If only 1, 2 and 3 are correct
    2 – If only 1 and 3 are correct
    3 – If only 2 and 4 are correct
    4 – If only 4 is correct
    5 – If all are correct

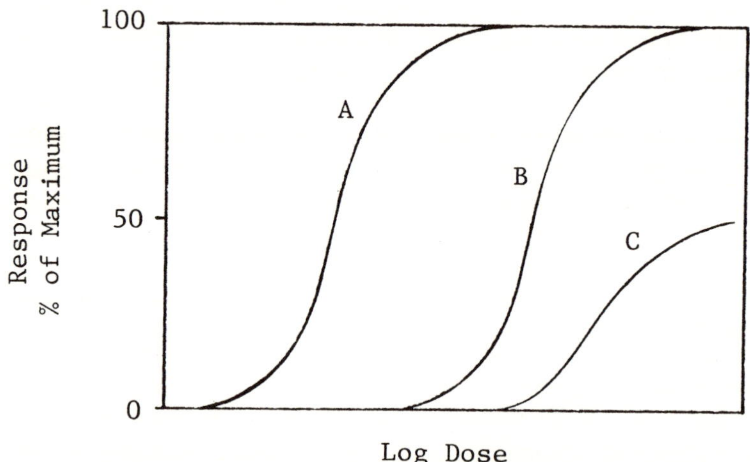

19. _______ Which of the following statements would be true concerning the above
curves?

    1. Curves A and B represent dose-response curves to two agonists
        which differ in their apparent affinity for the drug receptor
    2. Curve A represents the dose-response curve to an agonist and
        curve B represents the dose-response curve to the same agonist in
        the presence of a non-competitive inhibitor
    3. Curve A represents the dose-response curve to an agonist and
        curve B represents the dose-response curve to the same agonist in
        the presence of a competitive inhibitor
    4. Curves A and C represent dose-response curves to two agonists
        which have similar mechanisms of action because they are both
        producing the same pharmacological effect

20. _______ Which of the following statements are applicable to the absorption of
drugs after intramuscular administration?

    1. Absorption is slow because the drug does <u>not</u> diffuse over a large
        surface area
    2. Absorption is rapid compared with subcutaneous injection because
        the blood flow to skeletal muscle is large relative to
        subcutaneous tissues
    3. Lipoid solubility of the drug plays a major factor in the rate of
        absorption from this site
    4. Absorption can be delayed by administering the drug as an
        insoluble salt in suspension

<u>MULTIPLE TRUE-FALSE</u>
Directions Summarized:

1	2	3	4	5
1,2,3	1,3	2,4	4	all are
only	only	only	only	correct

21. _______ Which of the following statements are true of the binding of drugs to plasma protein?

    1. Bound drug acts as a storage site and can prolong the therapeutic effect if the drug is not eliminated by active processes
    2. Both free and bound drug are readily filtered by the kidney glomerulus
    3. A drug bound more than 90% to plasma albumin may require a priming dose to obtain a rapid therapeutic effect
    4. Only drugs which are weak acids, and not those which are weak bases, are bound to plasma protein

22. _______ Which of the following would be true of a drug which is eliminated from the body by processes exhibiting zero order kinetics?

    1. A constant amount of the drug is lost per unit time
    2. A constant percentage of the drug is lost per unit time
    3. This type of elimination indicates saturation of a transport process of depletion of a necessary cofactor
    4. With a constant dose and dosage interval, a plateau plasma concentration will be attained after 10-15 doses

23. _______ Which of the following are applicable to the conjugation of drugs with glucuronic acid?

    1. The enzymes mediating this reaction are located in the mitochondrial fraction of the liver
    2. The reaction requires prior activation of glucose to UDP-glucose and then oxidation to UDP-glucuronate
    3. Glucuronyl transferase activity is not increased by the chronic administration of phenobarbital
    4. The activity of glucuronyl transferase is low in new-borns and this observation is a potential explanation for the greater toxicity of some drugs in infants

<u>MULTIPLE TRUE-FALSE</u>
Directions Summarized:

1	2	3	4	5
1,2,3	1,3	2,4	4	all are
only	only	only	only	correct

24. _______ A drug is cleared from the plasma into the urine. The clearance value is 130 ml/min and the volume of distribution of the drug is 130 liters. Which of the following statements would be applicable to this drug?

1. The drug is excreted by both glomerular filtration and active tubular secretion
2. The drug is rapidly metabolized by the hepatic drug metabolizing system
3. The first order rate constant for excretion of the drug (K_e) is .1/min
4. The drug may be stored in a depot such as adipose tissue or cellular nucleic acids

25. _______ Which of the following statements can be applied to drug metabolism?

1. Metabolism of a drug may result in a product as active or more active than the parent compound
2. Metabolism of a drug can always be equated with inactivation or detoxication of the drug
3. The products of drug metabolism are generally more polar than the parent drug
4. All of the enzymes which have been associated with drug metabolism are found in the hepatic endoplasmic retuculum

26. _______ Glucuronide conjugation:

1. Is a highly developed protective mechanism of the newborn against foreign toxic compounds
2. Is a mechanism of detoxication of bilirubin as well as foreign compounds
3. Requires cytochrome P-450 for transfer of glucuronide to a drug
4. Is inducible by drugs such as phenobarbital

27. _______ Characteristics of the microsomal drug oxidizing system include:

1. The products of this system are usually less lipid soluble than are the substrates
2. Certain drugs and carcinogens may stimulate the activity of this system, probably as the result of <u>de novo</u> syntheis of the enzymes involved
3. The system is found primarily in the liver
4. The products of metabolism by this system are always pharmacologically less active than the substrates

<u>MULTIPLE TRUE-FALSE</u>
<u>Directions Summarized:</u>

1	2	3	4	5
1,2,3	1,3	2,4	4	all are
only	only	only	only	correct

28. _______ A drug may undergo little or no metabolic transformation in the body because:

1. It offers no site for drug-metabolizing enzymes to react with it
2. It is so highly ionized as to be inaccessible to intracellular sites of drug metabolism
3. It is strongly bound to plasma protein or intracellular binding sites
4. It fails to induce drug oxidation in hepatic endoplasmic reticulum

29. _______ Which of the following statements are applicable to the hepatic microsomal drug metabolizing enzymes?

1. Oxidations produced by this system require both NADPH and molecular oxygen
2. Transfer of oxygen to a drug molecule requires cytochrome P-450
3. The activity of this system can be increased by chronic administration of many lipid soluble compounds such as phenobarbital and methylcholanthrene
4. Microsomal preparations can also reduce susceptible drug substrates and the reduction may be mediated by either flavoprotein or cytochrome P-450

30. _______ Long persistence of a drug in the body may be associated with:

1. High lipoid solubility
2. Large volume of distribution
3. Low rate of excretion
4. Low rate of metabolism

31. _______ Which of the following metabolic pathways are catalyzed by cytochrome P-450?

1. The N-demethylation of diazepam
2. Metabolic activation of an aromatic carcinogen through an epoxide intermediate
3. Biosynthesis of cortisol
4. Glucuronidation of bilirubin

32. _______ Administration of phenobarbital would induce which of the following microsomal enzyme activities?

1. Sulfotransferase
2. Glucuronyl transferase
3. Cholinesterase
4. Phenytoin hydroxylase

MULTIPLE TRUE-FALSE
Directions Summarized:

1	2	3	4	5
1,2,3 only	1,3 only	2,4 only	4 only	all are correct

33. _______ The blood-brain barrier:

1. Restricts the entry of hydrophilic compounds into the brain
2. Has as one component, endothelial cells with pores accessible only by compounds of less than 200 daltons
3. Is between the plasma space and the interstitial space of the brain
4. Is not penetrated by organic solvents other than those used as anesthetic agents

34. _______ Covalent binding of drugs to body constituents:

1. May occur with competitive-irreversible antagonists
2. Occurs with all chemotherapeutic agents
3. May account for the hematopoietic toxicity of some drugs
4. Occurs because of the formation of strong Van der Waals forces

35. _______ Drug-receptor interactions:

1. Generally show kinetics like those for enzyme-substrate interactions
2. Occur only in the cell cytosol
3. Consist of both hydrophobic and ionic interactions in most cases
4. Can easily be identified by the use of radio-labelled agonists without taking the drug effect into consideration

36. _______ Transduction of drug binding to a receptor into a response might involve:

1. Changes in calcium gating in the membrane
2. Release into the cytosol of inositol triphosphate
3. Activation of adenylate cyclase by guanine nucleotide binding protein
4. Transport of complex from cytosol to nucleus

37. _______ Absorption of a drug from its site of administration:

1. Is slow for insoluble complexes
2. Is more rapid with increased blood flow
3. Is generally greater for more lipid soluble drugs
4. Is mainly influenced by the ionic state of the drug when the site is intramuscular or subcutaneous

<u>MULTIPLE TRUE-FALSE</u>
Directions Summarized:

1	2	3	4	5
1,2,3	1,3	2,4	4	all are
only	only	only	only	correct

38. _______ Drug bound to plasma protein:

    1. Might be bound to albumin if it is an acidic drug
    2. Might be bound to an α_1-acid glycoprotein if it is a basic drug
    3. Might be displaced from its binding site if a drug with a higher affinity for the site is given concurrently
    4. Always prolongs the duration of action of the drug

39. _______ Diminished response of an organ following continued application of a drug:

    1. Might result from the modification of a receptor so that it does not bind agonists
    2. Is called tachyphalaxis when it occurs rapidly
    3. Might result from the internalization of drug-receptor complexes
    4. Is an essential aspect of the theory involving spare receptors

40. _______ Termination of drug action:

    1. Can occur with elimination
    2. Always occurs with metabolism
    3. May involve redistribution of the drug in the body
    4. Is more rapid if the clearance of drug from blood is a small number

41. _______ Dose-dependent kinetics:

    1. Is another word for first-order kinetics
    2. Result because a pathway of elimination or excretion becomes saturated
    3. Has the same biologic half-life irrespective of the plasma drug concentration
    4. Indicate that a constant amount of drug is being lost per unit time

42. _______ Alteration of drug dosage schedule in a patient with kidney disease:

    1. Is more easily done than in patients with hepatic disease
    2. Generally is done using changes in creatinine clearance
    3. Is generally important if the drug is excreted more than 50% unchanged by the kidney
    4. The initial dose given the patient is not changed

<u>MULTIPLE TRUE-FALSE</u>
Directions Summarized:

1	2	3	4	5
1,2,3	1,3	2,4	4	all are
only	only	only	only	correct

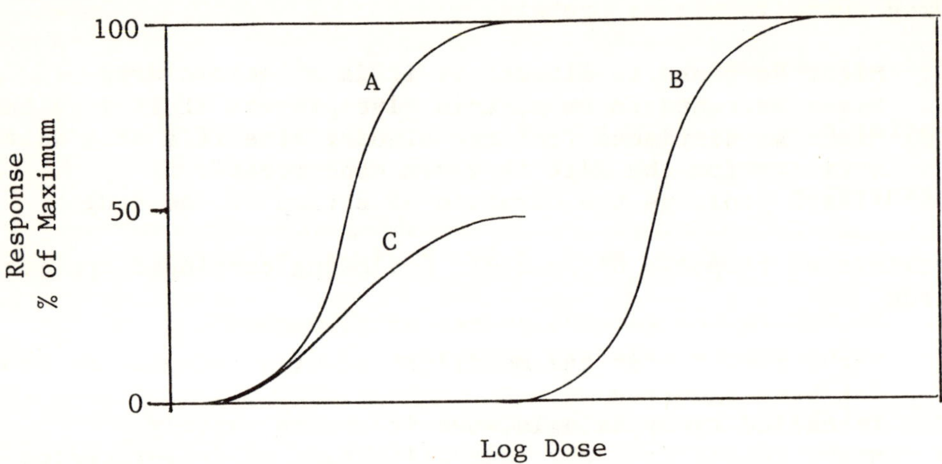

43. _______ Drugs A, B and C act on the same receptor. Which of the following
statements are applicable?

1. Drug A is a full agonist
2. Drug C is a full agonist
3. Drug B is a full agonist
4. Drug B is more potent than Drug A

44. _______ Referring to the same graph in question 43, which of the following
statements are applicable?

1. Curve B might be the response to Drug A in the presence of a
competitive inhibitor
2. Curve C might be the response to Drug A in the presence of a
noncompetitive inhibitor
3. The intrinsic activity of Drug C is less than that of Drug A
4. Mixtures of Drug A and Drug C would give curves showing
inhibition of the effects of A at high concentrations of C

MATCHING

1. Malignant hyperthemia with muscular rigidity
2. Atypical pseudocholinesterase
3. Glucose-6-phosphate dehydrogenase deficiency
4. Increased receptor affinity for menadione

45. _______ Halothane

46. _______ Succinylcholine

47. _______ Warfarin

48. _______ Primaquine

* * * * * * * * * *

1. Receptors for catecholamines or glucagon
2. Receptors for steroid hormones
3. Both
4. Neither

49. _______ Occur only in the endoplasmic reticulum and mediate changes in the amount of cytochrome P-450

50. _______ Coupled either in adenylate cyclase or to processes mediating calcium ion flux

ANSWERS

1.   __3__ $LD_{50} = T.I.; \dfrac{800}{ED_{50}} = \dfrac{1600}{200}$

2.   __1__   For Drug B, the dose-response curves for effectiveness and lethality overlap, which does not occur for Drug A.

3.   __1__   The ED_{50} for A is lower than that for B.

4.   __2__   Answer 1 is a misstatement, it should be increased transiently rather than decreased. 3 - Filtration at the glomerulus is directly related to free drug in the plasma. 4 - The priming dose is used to compensate for protein binding which doesn't occur to as great an extent in the presence of X. 5-This is a "classic" drug interaction relative to protein binding.

5.   __5__   All are correct. It is usually implicit that half-life values relate to drugs eliminated by first order kinetics. 3 and 4 are statements applicable to any drug.

6.   __5__   1 to 3 are involved in conjugation mechanisms. Oxidation requires NADPH, oxygen and cytochrome P-450.

7.   __2__

8.   __5__

9.   __2__   After conjugation, the ability of the drug to penetrate to sites of metabolism are decreased.

10.   __4__

11.   __3__

12.   __2__ X_0 can be calculated from the data given. $t_{\frac{1}{2}}$ is 4 hrs. Twice plasma concentration at 4 hrs is 4.8 μg/ml or 4.8 mg/L.

$$V.D. = \frac{dose}{X_0} = \frac{500}{4.8} = 100\ L$$

13.   __5__

$$t_{\frac{1}{2}} = 0.7\ \frac{V.D.}{clearance}$$

$$4\ hr = 0.7\ \frac{100\ L}{clearance}$$

$$Cl = \frac{70}{4} = \sim 18 L/hr = 300\ ml/min$$

This is greater than GFR but much less than renal plasma flow.

14.   __4__   Toxicity occurs at 4.5 μg/ml

$$Plasma\ concentration = \frac{infusion\ rate}{clearance}$$

$$= \frac{1.5\ mg/min}{300\ ml/min}$$

$$= .005\ mg/ml$$

$$= 5\ \mu g/ml$$

Toxicity occurs at 90% of this value. With drugs which follow first order kinetics, this value is reached in 3.3 half-lives or 3.3 x 4 = 13.2.

15.   __3__   Need to solve for dose in formula:

$$Plasma\ concentration = \frac{1.5\ (dose/interval)\ (t_{\frac{1}{2}})}{vol.\ distribution}$$

$$3.3\ \mu g/ml = \frac{1.5\ (D/8)\ (4)}{100L.}$$

$$3.3 = \frac{0.75D}{100}$$

$$= 440\ mg$$

16. __2__   Variation equal to dose divided by volume of distribution.
17. __3__
18. __4__
19. __2__   2 is incorrect because a non-competitive inhibitor would decrease the maximal response. 4 is incorrect because drugs with similar mechanisms of action produce parallel dose-response curves with similar maximal responses, although that is still not sufficient to prove same mechanism.
20. __3__   1 is incorrect because absorption is rapid and the surface area is large. 3 is incorrect because drugs can pass easily through spaces between endothelial cells in the capillaries or can go through the lymphatic system which at its ends in the muscle are openings without membranes.
21. __2__   2 is incorrect because only free drug is filtered. 4 is incorrect because strong acids and both strong and weak bases can be bound to plasma protein.
22. __2__   1 and 2 are mutually exclusive and 2 defines a first order process. 4 is incorrect because the time to reach a plateau concentration is dose-dependent and not readily predicted.
23. __3__   1 is incorrect because the localization is the microsomal fraction. 3 is incorrect because phenobarbital pretreatment increases this enzymic activity and has been used in attempts to treat some cases of hereditary hyperbilirubinemias.
24. __4__   1 is incorrect because the clearance value is not high enough to indicate active secretion. 2 is incorrect because the large value for the volume of distribution indicates binding to tissue constituents which limits presentation of the drug to sites of metabolism. 3 is incorrect because the calculated value is .001/min.
25. __2__   1 and 2 are mutually exclusive and 1 is correct. 4 is incorrect because the enzymes can occur in the cytosol or mitochondria as well as tissues other than the liver.
26. __3__   Newborns lack glucuronide conjugation and P-450 is not involved.
27. __1__
28. __1__   Induction is not a prerequisite for metabolism. Tight-binding to plasma protein will decrease metabolism but in some cases binding is associated with a more rapid clearance. This finding suggests an active transport into the liver cell.
29. __5__
30. __5__
31. __1__   Adrenal cortex utilizes cytochrome P-450 for biosynthesis
32. __3__
33. __1__   4 incorrect because all lipid soluble substances penetrate.
34. __2__
35. __2__   Have to have an effect
36. __5__
37. __1__
38. __1__   Drugs actively secreted are shortened in duration
39. __1__
40. __2__
41. __3__   Dose-dependent kinetics same as zero order kinetics
42. __5__
43. __2__   Drug C partial agonist   47. __4__
44. __5__   48. __3__
45. __1__   49. __4__
46. __2__   50. __1__

SECTION II: <u>AUTONOMIC DRUGS</u>

I. <u>SYMPATHETIC DIVISION</u> (Adrenergic)

    A. <u>Functional</u>

        1. Only major <u>tone</u> to blood vessels (<u>alpha</u>-adrenoceptors) – decrease BP due to decrease in sympathetic tone (also mechanism for baroreceptors). Heart rate and contractile force increased due to sympathetic activation – this is a unique action of norepinephrine (NE) acting on the <u>beta</u>$_1$ receptors.

        2. Eye: Dilated iris <u>via</u> sympathetic action on radial muscle.

        3. G.I. tract inhibited by sympathetics – both <u>alpha</u> and <u>beta</u> receptors. Bronchi dilated primarily by circulating epinephrine acting on <u>beta</u>$_2$ receptor.

        4. Sweat glands – part of sympathetic system but ACh is the transmitter at neuroeffector junction (sympathetic-cholinergic).

        5. Humoral effects of epinephrine include breakdown of glycogen (glycogenolysis) and free fatty acid release.

    B. <u>Synthesis and Termination</u> – Tyrosine converted by enzyme tyrosine hydroxylase to dopa. Dopa to dopamine and dopamine to norepinephrine via action of dopa decarboxylase and dopamine-<u>beta</u>-hydroxylase (in storage granule) respectively. (First two enzymes are cytoplasmic). Cytoplasmic enzyme in the adrenal medulla (phenylethanolamine-N-methyl-transferase) transfer of methyl group to form epinephrine. Norepinephrine and epinephrine have negative feedback action on activity of tyrosine hydroxylase. Termination of action is primarily by reuptake (60-90%) into nerve terminal. Secondary inactivation by MAO (primarily intraneuronal) and COMT (primarily extraneuronal). Both enzymes also in gut wall and liver.

    C. <u>Catecholamines</u> – must have 3,4-OH substitution on benzene ring. COMT acts here (primarily extraneuronal). <u>Alpha</u> carbon CH_3 substitution protects against MAO which acts primarily within the nerve terminal. Product of breakdown by <u>both</u> MAO and COMT = vanilmandelic acid (VMA); also called 3-methoxy-4-hydroxy-mandelic acid. This is one of compounds screened for in suspected pheochromocytoma.

        1. <u>Norepinephrine</u>: endogenous neurotransmitter (NE).

           a. Catecholamine released from all sympathetic nerves (except sympathetic-cholinergic system); <u>Tyrosine Hydroxylase</u> is rate limiting step in synthesis; acts strongly on <u>alpha</u> but not on <u>beta</u> receptors with <u>exception</u> of those in the heart. Direct acting and not effective orally (broken down by MAO and COMT in gut wall and liver).

           b. Stimulates <u>alpha</u> receptors (<u>alpha</u>$_1$ and <u>alpha</u>$_2$) in vascular smooth muscle; arterioles in skin and mucosa, splanchnic, renal and coronary vascular beds directly constricted; TPR, diastolic and systolic BP increases; veins also constricted; increased BP activates baroreceptors to reflexly increase vagal activity.

    c. Direct effect on <u>beta</u>$_1$ receptors of heart to increase heart rate, automaticity increased by increasing rate of slow diastolic (phase 4) depolarization and to increase force and velocity of contraction. Reflex vagal slowing of HR can oppose direct effects of NE and result in decreased output even though force and stroke volume is increased.

2. <u>Epinephrine</u> (Epi): endogenous catecholamine in adrenal medulla.
    a. About 90% of catecholamine released from adrenal medulla; is a hormone; acts strongly on <u>both</u> <u>alpha</u> and <u>beta</u> adrenergic receptors by a <u>direct</u> action; not effective orally; causes metabolic actions seen in fight or flight response.
    b. Epi stimulates both <u>alpha</u> and <u>beta</u>$_2$ receptors in blood vessels; with small doses or with slow infusion, get vasodilation (skeletal muscle) and diastolic BP decreases (<u>beta</u>$_2$ effect); with larger doses, get vasoconstriction (skin and splanchnics) and TPR is increased (<u>alpha</u> effect); veins are constricted.
    c. Direct effect on <u>beta</u>$_1$, receptor of heart – like NE; increased rate (automaticity), force and cardiac output; with large doses; acts like NE to cause reflex vagal slowing and decreased output despite direct effects.

3. <u>Isoproterenol</u>: synthetic <u>beta</u>-adrenoceptor stimulant.
    a. Also catecholamine; acts directly on all <u>beta</u> adrenergic receptors; no <u>alpha</u> action; not effective orally; used in treatment of asthma (<u>beta</u>$_2$) and experimentally in cardiogenic shock (<u>beta</u>$_1$).
    b. Stimulates <u>beta</u>$_2$ receptors of blood vessels to cause vasodilation – decreased diastolic BP and TPR.
    c. Direct <u>beta</u>$_1$ receptor stimulation in heart to increase rate, force and output; no reflex vagal activation.

4. <u>Dopamine</u> (DA):
    a. Catecholamine; precursor in formation of NE and E in peripheral autonomic system; probably acts as CNS neurotransmitter especially in extrapyramidal motor system.
    b. Not orally effective; acts on <u>alpha</u> and <u>beta</u>$_1$ receptors to increase BP and HR; also causes vasodilation of renal vasculature by action on "dopamine receptors".
    c. Sometimes used in treatment of patients with shock primarily for cardiac and renal actions.
    d. Replacement in CNS by giving precursor (ℓ-DOPA) is a principal treatment to relieve the symptoms of Parkinson's disease.

D. <u>Sympathomimetics</u> (Non-catecholamines) – May exert effects by direct or indirect actions. <u>Direct</u> sympathomimetics act to stimulate <u>alpha</u> or <u>beta</u>-adrenoceptors. <u>Indirect</u> sympathomimetics may release stored NE from nerve terminals or may block reuptake mechanism (many do both). <u>Tricyclic Antidepressants</u> act like <u>cocaine</u> in preventing reuptake of catecholamines into nerve terminals. <u>Reuptake</u> is principle mechanism for termination of the actions of NE. <u>Imipramine</u> and <u>amitriptyline</u>.

    1. <u>Tyramine</u>: indirect actions only – effects produced by the release of endogenous norepinephrine from storage granules; will be ineffective if animal pretreated with reserpine or chronically with guanethidine. Found in foods such as wine, cheese, beer, etc. but is normally broken down by MAO in gut (no <u>alpha</u>-carbon CH$_3$).

Tyramine in foods can lead to hypertensive crisis in patients on MAO inhibitor drugs such as pargyline and tranylcypromine; cardiovascular effects on heart and blood vessels produced by the NE released.

2 & 3. <u>Amphetamine</u> and <u>Methamphetamine</u>: indirect acting (primarily releases endogenous NE). Orally effective due to <u>alpha</u> carbon CH_3 group. Potent CNS effects. Tolerance readily develops to appetite supressive and mood elevating effects. Causes syndrome resembling paranoia in repeated large doses; only slight direct action on peripheral <u>alpha</u> receptors. Acidification of urine with ammonium chloride aids in renal elimination.

STRUCTURES AND MAIN CLINICAL USES OF SOME IMPORTANT SYMPATHOMIMETIC DRUGS

		β CH	α CH	NH	ACTION	α-RECEPTOR A,N,P,V	β-RECEPTOR B,C	CNS
Phenylethylamine		H	H	H				
Epinephrine	3-OH, 4-OH	OH	H	CH_3	DIRECT	A,P,V	B,C	
Norepinephrine	3-OH, 4-OH	OH	H	H	DIRECT	P		
Isoproterenol	3-OH, 4-OH	OH	H	$CH(CH_3)_2$	DIRECT		B,C	
Dopamine	3-OH, 4-OH	H	H	H	DIRECT	P	C	CNS
Tyramine	4-OH	H	H	H	INDIRECT			
Amphetamine		H	CH_3	H	INDIRECT			CNS
Phenylpropanolamine		OH	CH_3	H	INDIRECT			CNS
Methamphetamine		H	CH_3	CH_3	INDIRECT	P		CNS
Ephedrine		OH	CH_3	CH_3	MIXED	N,P	B,C	
Metaraminol	3-OH	OH	CH_3	H	DIRECT	P		
Phenylephrine	3-OH	OH	H	CH_3	DIRECT	N,P		
Methoxamine	2-OCH_3, 5-OCH_3	OH	CH_3	H	DIRECT	P		
Metaproterenol	3-OH, 5-OH	OH	H	$CH(CH_3)_2$	DIRECT		B	
Terbutaline	3-OH, 5-OH	OH	H	$C(CH_3)_3$	DIRECT		B	
Albuterol	3-CH_2OH, 4-OH	OH	H	$C(CH_3)_3$	DIRECT		B	
Ritodrine	4-OH	OH	CH_3	1	DIRECT		U,B	
Dobutamine	3-OH, 4-OH	H	H	2	DIRECT		C	

A: Allergic reactions
N: Nasal decongestion
P: Pressor (may include   action)
V: Local vasoconstriction
     (e.g. in local anesthetics)
B: Bronchodilator
C: Cardiac
U: Uterine relaxant
CNS: Central nervous system

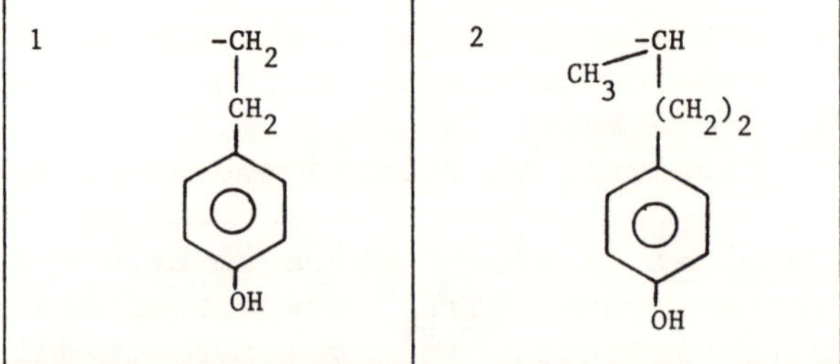

4. <u>Phenylpropanolamine</u>: many actions same as amphetamine; orally effective; anorexiant action questionable; occasional use as nasal decongestant. Note that drugs that are without 3- or 4-OH on ring and with CH_3 on <u>alpha</u>-carbon are refractory to breakdown by MAO and COMT.

5. <u>Ephedrine</u>: mixed actions (direct and indirect) acts like epinephrine on both <u>alpha</u> and <u>beta</u> receptors; orally effective; one of most commonly used sympathomimetics; increases BP, heart rate

and contractility; bronchial muscle relaxation; mydriasis without cycloplegia.

6. <u>Metaraminol</u>: mixed acting; more direct than indirect and mainly acts on <u>alpha</u> receptors. May cause hypotension if given over long periods of time as is taken into nerve terminals where it can serve as a false transmitter. Used to elevate BP in hypotensive states.

7. <u>Phenylephrine</u>: direct acting - primarily on <u>alpha</u> receptors; oral dose much greater than i.v. or i.m. dose; widely used as nasal decongestant but can lead to more congestion via irritant actions on nasal mucosa (rebound phenomena); produces vasoconstriction with minimal cardiac effects. Sometimes used to treat paroxysmal atrial tachycardia (PAT).

8. <u>Methoxamine</u>: direct acting - like phenylephrine; vasoconstrictor; almost pure <u>alpha</u> with minimal cardiac effects; as above may use to treat PAT; no significant CNS effects.

9. <u>Metaproterenol</u>: direct acting; "selective" B_2 agonist; used as bronchodilator with minimal cardiac actions; orally effective (resistant to COMT); sometimes used to inhibit uterus in premature labor.

10. <u>Terbutaline</u>: direct acting; also "selective" B_2 agonist; used as bronchodilator; uses and actions similar to metaproterenol. Oral, s.c. or inhalation, longer acting than metaproterenol but more cardiac effects.

11. <u>Albuterol</u>: similar indications to terbutaline; inhalation or oral; duration similar to metaproterenol; few CV effects.

12. <u>Ritodrine</u>: <u>Beta</u>$_2$ selective; developed as a uterine relaxant; 30% absorbed by oral route; administered also IV and IM.

13. <u>Dobutamine</u>: direct acting; "selective" B_1 agonist; used to increase heart rate and contractility; increases myocardial contractile force more than HR; short acting and not orally effective; given as i.v. infusion. Used to treat congestive heart failure.

E. <u>Drugs Inhibiting Sympathetic Function</u> (Sympatholytics)

1. <u>False Transmitter Precursors</u>:
   a. <u>Alpha methyl meta tyrosine</u> → metaraminol
   b. <u>alpha methyl dopa</u> → <u>alpha methyl NE</u> (CNS action in treating hypertension).

2. <u>MAO inhibitors</u>:
   a. <u>Pargyline</u> and <u>tranylcypromine</u>; <u>toxic</u> as also inhibit other enzyme systems; CNS effects may be related to increased levels of NE in brain; MAO also is enzyme responsible for breakdown of serotonin (5-HT). May cause hypotension as <u>intraneuronal</u> tyrosine can be changed to tyramine and then to octopamine (false transmitter).

3. <u>Adrenergic Neuron Inhibitors</u>:
   a. <u>Reserpine</u>: prevents storage and thus causes depletion of neuronal NE. Also depletes stores of epinephrine, dopamine and serotonin; CNS effects include sedation.
   b. <u>Guanethidine</u>: blocks nerve action potentials at fine terminals (also has many other actions). Effective and potent antihypertensive drug; orally effective; does not act on CNS; chronic administration also depletes <u>peripheral</u> catecholamine.

Taken up by nerve endings, thus effect blocked by reuptake inhibitors (tricyclics and cocaine).

4. <u>Alpha Receptor Blockers</u>: side effects include postural hypotension (orthostatic), reflex tachycardia, miosis, nasal stuffiness, inhibition of ejaculation.

   a. <u>Phenoxybenzamine</u> – specific blockade of <u>alpha</u> receptors and vasoconstriction caused by nerve stimulation or sympathomimetic drugs; produces fall in BP by reducing sympathetic tone, but get tachycardia because <u>beta</u> receptors not blocked; causes Epi "reversal" – converts a pressor response to Epi to a depressor response (no effect on cardiostimulation to Epi); longer acting agent; first competitive then becomes noncompetitive. Used during treatment of pheochromocytoma.

   b. <u>Phentolamine</u>: short acting due only to competive blockade of <u>alpha</u> receptors; used in diagnosis of pheochromocytoma (Regitine Test); also releases histamine leading to false positive tests; used to block excessive pressor rise caused by catecholamines released by pheochromocytoma during surgical removal; blocks $alpha_1$ and $alpha_2$ receptors.

   c. <u>Prazosin</u>: used in treatment of hypertension, probably due to blockade of peripheral $alpha_1$ adrenoceptors; may have some direct vasodilator action; less reflex tachycardia observed which may be due to the agent's selective blockade of $alpha_1$ adrenergic receptors (allowing for the negative feedback of $alpha_2$ presynaptic mechanism in the heart); may have CNS effect to decrease sympathetic tone.

   d. <u>Yohimbine</u>: "selective" antagonist for $alpha_2$ adrenoceptors; experimentally shown to antagonize CNS hypotensive actions of clonidine and <u>alpha</u>-methyl-DOPA.

5. <u>Beta Receptor Blockers</u>: used to treat hypertension, angina, cardiac arrhythmias, reduce incidence of myocardial reinfarction. Caution in patients with congestive heart failure, bronchial asthma, or diabetes.

   a. <u>Propranolol</u>: nonselective <u>beta</u> receptor antagonist (blocks both $beta_1$ and $beta_2$ receptors); orally effective; $t_{\frac{1}{2}}$ = 3-5 hrs., first-pass hepatic metabolism seen particularly with the initial dose; 90% bound to plasma proteins; has a local anesthetic ("quinidine like") action; used in treating cardiac arrhythmias and in treating hypertension. Use with caution especially in patients with heart disease, asthma and diabetes (may mask the tachycardia "sign" of hypoglycemia).

   b. <u>Metoprolol</u>: cardio-selective $beta_1$ adrenergic antagonist (50X more potent for $beta_1$); like propranolol, subject to first-pass metabolic breakdown by liver; only slight membrane stabilizing action; 10% bound to plasma proteins; less effect on bronchial smooth muscle; more CNS side effects.

   c. <u>Atenolol</u>: Also cardioselective ($beta_1$); longer half life (6-9 hrs) thus fewer doses needed; renal excretion; less hypoglycemia and less CNS effects.

   d. <u>Pindolol</u>: nonselective; hepatic and renal elimination; intrinsic sympathomimetic activity (ISA) may contribute to less depression of HR and CO at rest.

   e. <u>Nadolol</u>: also nonselective <u>beta</u> receptor antagonist; longer acting than propranolol ($t_{\frac{1}{2}}$ = 20-24 hrs), thus suitable for once per day administration; no significant local anesthetic or "quinidine-like" action; no ISA; excluded from CNS.

    f. **Timolol**: non-selective **beta** receptor antagonist; no significant local anesthetic or "quinidine-like" action; 5 to 10X as potent as propranolol; a drug of choice given topically to treat open angle glaucoma (reduces formation of aqueous humor); also used post- myocardial infarction.

6. **Mixed Antagonist**:

    a. **Labetalol**: **Alpha**$_1$ antagonist; nonselective **beta**-antagonist; some **beta**$_2$-stimulation. Oral or i.v.; t½ about 5 hrs; decreases plasma renin. Used to treat hypertension and sometimes clonidine withdrawal syndrome. Postural hypotension (**alpha**) and other side effects as with **beta** antagonists.

II. PARASYMPATHETIC DIVISION (Cholinergic)

A. Functional

1. Bradycardia via efferent vagus; little or no direct action on contractile force. No parasympathetic tone to blood vessels in general.
2. Eye: main tone to iris; causes miosis upon stimulation – involvement in light reflex – also tone to ciliary body. Blockade leads to mydriasis and cycloplegia; overactivity leads to miosis and spasm of accomodation.
3. Constriction of bronchial tree – of little significance in man; increased tone of G.I. tract and urinary bladder; increased G.I. secretions.
4. Parasympathetic stimulation of salivary glands → profuse, watery saliva. Parotid gland innervated only by parasympathetic system.
5. **Botulinus toxin**: prevents release of ACh; **Hemicholinium**: prevents reuptake of choline; **Black Widow spider venom**: causes excessive release of ACh.
6. Acetyl–CoA + Choline → Acetylcholine; enzyme is choline acetylase. ACh stored in granules; breakdown rapid via specific enzyme called acetylcholinesterase.

B. Synthesis and Termination of Effect – synthesized by enzyme choline acetyltransferase (choline acetylase) by complexing choline with acetyl coenzyme A to produce acetylcholine. Destruction of acetylcholine is by cholinesterases to produce acetic acid and choline. Acetylcholinesterases located in neuronal membranes and red blood cells; pseudocholinesterase (non-specific or butyrylcholinesterase) more widely distributed.

C. Choline Esters

1. **Acetylcholine**: endogenous neurotransmitter (ACh).

    a. Acts on nicotinic and muscarinic receptors (all parasympathetic end organs; autonomic ganglia; NMJ; adrenal medulla; some sympathetic nerves to skeletal muscle blood vessels and to sweat glands; CNS muscarinic and nicotinic receptors).

    b. The smooth muscle of blood vessels is directly relaxed by small doses of ACh which stimulate **muscarinic** cholinergic receptors; decreases TPR, mean and diastolic BP; the drop in BP will elicit

<u>via</u> the baroreceptor mechanism a reflex increase of sympathetic activity.

    c. Direct effects on cardiac <u>muscarinic</u> cholinergic receptors to decrease heart rate (automaticity decreased by decreasing rate of slow diastolic (phase 4) depolarization) and to decrease contractile force; speeds conduction of electrical impulses in atrial muscle but slows conduction through the AV node and prolongs refractory period of the AV node; reflex sympathetic activity to speed HR and increase cardiac contractility will oppose direct ACh actions on the heart.

2. <u>Methacholine</u>: ACh with CH_3 substitution; strong muscarinic action; little nicotinic effects; partially refractory to enzyme hydrolysis; following i.v. administration BP falls greatly (blocked by atropine).

3. <u>Carbachol</u>: ACh plus terminal NH_2; strong nicotinic action; lesser muscarinic actions; almost totally refractory to hydrolysis (following atropine, BP increases); also releases ACh.

4. <u>Bethanechol</u>: CH_3 and NH_2 addition to ACh; ester of choice in treatment of urinary retention and to increase G.I. motility. Has both muscarinic and nicotinic actions; refractory to enzyme breakdown.

E. <u>Cholinomimetic Alkaloids</u>

1. <u>Muscarine</u>: classical agent – in part responsible for rapid type of mushroom poisoning; acts strongly on all muscarinic receptors; hypotension; glandular secretions.

2. <u>Pilocarpine</u>: muscarinic stimulant; a drug of choice in treatment of glaucoma (contracts ciliary muscle and constricts pupil).

3. <u>Nicotine</u>: isolated from tobacco leaves; nicotinic receptor stimulant; colorless liquid in pure state; activation of NMJ, all ganglia; adrenal medulla.

F. <u>Cholinergic Blocking Agents</u>

1. <u>Atropine</u>: prototype; strongly blocks muscarinic receptors. Selective competitive block of muscarinic receptors; also has prominent CNS effects; low doses may slow HR by central action; larger doses will increase HR and speed conduction of impulses through the AV node; cardiac contractility usually unaffected except at very high dosages which can depress contractility. At very high doses, generalized vasodilation also may occur because of depressant effects; at low doses causes vascular muscle in blush area to relax but no prominent effects on pressure; low doses will block responses to nerve stimulation or injected cholinergic drugs; decreased G.I. and urinary bladder motility, lack of sweating and dry mouth. Little direct effect on B.P. Frequently used as preanesthetic medication. Very toxic in children; treat with physostigmine; dangerous in glaucoma patients.

2. <u>Scopolamine</u>: like atropine blocks all muscarinic receptors; in adults may cause more sedation than atropine.

3. <u>Homatropine Methylbromide</u>: has N^+ group; used orally for local action on G.I. tract.

4. <u>Atropine Substitutes</u>: many quaternary ammonium or tertiary amino derivatives synthesized; all closely resemble natural alkaloid; many

      used in ophthalmology to produce mydriasis and cycloplegia due to shorter duration of action.

5. <u>Benztropine</u>: stronger CNS effect; less peripheral action; used in treatment of Parkinson's disease.

G. <u>Anticholinesterase Agents</u> – enhance cholinergic function by complexing with enzyme that breaks down ACh (acetylcholinesterase). Signs and symptoms include activation of nicotinic and muscarinic receptors.

1. <u>Physostigmine</u>: also called eserine, acts only as an anti-AChase. Effects last 4 to 6 hrs.; rarely used clinically as other drugs are better due to dual action (see below). Rational use would include treatment of atropine poisoning due to entry into CNS. Binds to both sites on enzyme.

2. <u>Neostigmine</u>: acts as physostigmine but also has direct action on skeletal muscle; one drug of choice in treatment of myasthenia gravis; 4-6 hr action; binds to both anionic and ester sites on enzyme.

3. <u>Pyridostigmine</u> and <u>ambenonium</u>: used in treatment of myasthenia gravis especially in patients that have become tolerant to actions of neostigmine. Actions and binding are similar.

4. <u>Edrophonium</u>: short acting; binds strongly only to anionic enzyme site. Useful in diagnosis of myasthenia gravis and "cholinergic crisis".

5. <u>Parathion and Isoflurophate (D.F.P.)</u>: "nonreversible" as are very slowly released from enzyme by hydrolysis; bind to ester site on enzyme. Are used primarily as insecticides; some used topically to treat glaucoma. Can be removed from enzyme by oxime reactivators such as <u>2-PAM</u> (pralidoxime) along with atropine (for muscarinic effects).

III. <u>AUTONOMIC GANGLIA</u>

ACh released at ganglionic synapse.
Adrenal medulla – pharmacologically behaves as a sympathetic ganglion and is stimulated and blocked by agents acting on autonomic ganglia.

A. <u>Ganglionic Stimulants</u>

1. <u>General Action</u>: stimulates all autonomic ganglia, both sympathetic and parasympathetic. Unique drugs, both stimulants and blockers (dose dependent effects) of autonomic ganglia. Experimental interest – no therapeutic uses – stimulate ganglion cells directly.

2. <u>Agents</u>:
Nicotine (small dose)
TMA (tetramethylammonium)
DMPP
Acetylcholine (large doses)

3. <u>Actions</u>:
<u>Cardiovascular (primarily due to sympathetic stimulation)</u>; vasoconstriction, tachycardia, blood pressure elevation, cardiac force and output increased; (<u>secondary-parasympathetic and reflex effects ensue</u>); slowing of heart rate, brief episodes of vagal arrest with escape; cardiac arrhythmias due to imbalance of vagal slowing (mediated <u>via</u> ACh release) vs. increased sympathetic

activity (mediated <u>via</u> catecholamine release) to enhance automaticity.

B. <u>Ganglionic Blocking Drugs</u>

1. <u>General Action</u>: blockade and inhibition of transmission at both sympathetic and parasympathetic ganglia.
2. <u>Agents</u>:
   a. <u>Hexamethonium</u> (C_6) and <u>Tetraethylammonium</u> (TEA): short acting; N+ group therefore not effective orally.
   b. <u>Chlorisondamine</u> and <u>Mecamylamine</u>: longer acting; orally effective.
   c. <u>Trimethaphan</u>: only agent used today with any frequency; used in surgery to reduce B.P.; ultra short acting = rapid recovery.
   d. <u>d-Tubocurarine</u>: also blocks ganglia at moderate to high concentrations.
   e. <u>Nicotine</u>: large or repeated doses produce depolarization blockade.
3. <u>Effects of ganglionic blockade include</u>:
   a. Decreased blood pressure due to decreased sympathetic tone.
   b. Tachycardia or bradycardia depending on heart rate prior to blockade.
   c. Mydriasis and cycloplegia (dilated pupil and paralysis of accommodation).
   d. Decreased G. I. and urinary tone; dry mouth (xerostomia) and lack of sweating (anhidrosis); dry mouth overcome by muscarinic stimulants such as pilocarpine.
   e. Postural hypotension: reflex adjustments blocked; vasodilation, hypotension, increased peripheral flow, pooling of blood, decreased venous return, and decreased output.

IV. <u>NEUROMUSCULAR BLOCKING DRUGS</u>

A. <u>Functional</u>

1. Depression of neuromuscular function:
   <u>Tetrodotoxin</u> – blocks Na^+ conductance; <u>Batrachotoxin</u> – increases K^+ conductance; <u>Hemicholinium</u> – inhibits choline uptake for synthesis; <u>Botulinus toxin</u> – binds to sites on prejunctional membrane and prevents release of ACh; <u>Black Widow Spider toxin</u> – clumping of vesicles at prejunctional membrane, thus excessive release followed by depression; <u>antibiotics</u> (neomycin, streptomycin, etc.) depress ACh release; <u>general anesthetics</u> – stabilize membrane, thus inhibit response by ACh; lack of Ca^{++}; snake <u>alpha</u>-toxins bind irreversibly to receptors.
2. Facilitation of neuromuscular function: excess Ca^{++}; catecholamines; anticholinesterase agents (i.e., neostigmine, physostigmine, etc.); K^+ ion.

B. <u>Competitive Agents</u> – compete with acetylcholine for postjunctional receptors at endplate; blockade overcome by anticholinesterase drugs.

1. <u>d-Tubocurarine</u>: produces flaccid paralysis lasting from 10 to 40 minutes; smaller muscles affected first, diaphragm last. Effects potentiated by 1) anesthetics (ether, halothane, cyclopropane, and methoxyflurane), and 2) antibiotics (neomycin, streptomycin,

kanamycin, etc.). Effects can be reversed by anticholinesterase agents (i.e., neostigmine and edrophonium). Hypotension is observed and is caused by both release of <u>histamine</u> and ganglionic blockade. No CNS effects. Not analgesic. Myasthenia gravis patients are very sensitive to these agents. Bronchospasm may occur due to histamine release. Mainly metabolized; can be excreted in bile. Also release heparin.

2. <u>Metocurine</u>: methylation of —OH groups; 3 times as potent as curare; actions similar to curare.

3. <u>Pancuronium</u>: like above but more potent and much less release of histamine; steroid nucleus. Excreted in urine, thus may create problem in patients with kidney disease.

4. <u>Gallamine</u>: shorter duration than d-tubocurarine; causes selective cardiac vagal blockade. In other respects like pancuronium; no histamine or ganglionic blockade. Contraindicated in cardiac and renal disease.

5. <u>Atricurium</u>: short acting due to spontaneous degradation at physiological pH; about same potency as curare; less histamine release; no CV side effects. Especially suited for patients with impaired hepatic or renal function.

6. <u>Vecuronium</u>: more potent analog of pancuronium; shorter duration due to enhanced metabolism; suitable in patients with renal failure; no significant ganglionic or vagal blockade.

C. <u>Depolarizing Agents</u> – produce initial depolarization of endplate (phase i) which over time may develop into a "receptor inactivation" block (phase ii). Anticholinergic agents enhance blockade.

1. <u>Succinylcholine</u>: short acting; used for shorter procedures; also releases histamine and blocks ganglia. Produces initial fasciculations of muscle and blockade is potentiated by anticholinesterase agents. Broken down by plasma and liver pseudocholinesterase, therefore can cause problems in patients with low levels of this enzyme. Also competes with procaine, etc., for enzyme sites. Can cause an increase in intraoccular pressure and cerebrospinal fluid pressure. May trigger "malignant hyperthermia".

2. <u>Decamethonium (C-10)</u>: similar to succinylcholine, but longer duration of action; not used clinically.

REVIEW QUESTIONS

<u>ONE BEST ANSWER</u>

1. _______ All of the following compounds are precursors of norepinephrine and epinephrine in the body EXCEPT:

    1. 3,4 Dihydroxyphenylethylamine (Dopamine)
    2. Phenylalanine
    3. Tyrosine
    4. 3,4 Dihydroxyphenylalanine (DOPA)
    5. 3-Methoxy, 4-hydroxy mandelic acid (VMA)

2. _______ Adrenergic <u>beta</u> receptors subserve all of the following actions EXCEPT:

    1. Vasodilation
    2. Bronchodilation
    3. Increased myocardial contractile force
    4. Contraction of the radial muscle of the iris
    5. Increased heart rate

3. _______ With which of the following conditions would atropine most likely be contraindicated?

    1. Myasthenia gravis
    2. Asthma
    3. Glaucoma
    4. Nasal congestion
    5. Hypertension

4. _______ Bronchial asthma is an indication for all of the following EXCEPT:

    1. Epinephrine
    2. Ephedrine
    3. Carbachol
    4. Corticosteroids
    5. Aminophylline

5. _______ The drug of first choice in the emergency treatment of anaphylactic shock is:

    1. Epinephrine
    2. Norepinephrine
    3. Cortisone
    4. Diphenhydramine
    5. Atropine

<u>ONE BEST ANSWER</u>

6. _______ All of the following constrict bronchiolar smooth muscle EXCEPT:

    1. Serotonin
    2. Histamine
    3. Acetylcholine
    4. Bradykinin
    5. Theophylline

7. _______ Succinylcholine is hydrolyzed to succinic acid and choline by the action of which one of the following?

    1. Acetylcholine
    2. Anticholinesterase
    3. Non-specific plasma cholinesterase
    4. Choline acetylase

8. _______ In a patient receiving atropine, norepinephrine produces an increased blood pressure and heart rate. After this patient has been given an unknown drug, the administration of norepinephrine now produces about the same increase in heart rate as it did previously but a smaller increase in blood pressure. The unknown drug could be:

    1. Reserpine
    2. Propranolol
    3. Guanethidine
    4. Phenoxybenzamine
    5. Hexamethonium

9. _______ The therapeutic effectiveness of neostigmine in myasthenia gravis is thought to be due to:

    1. Its ability to protect the muscle end plate against acetylcholine
    2. Its ability to increase the rate of synthesis of acetylcholine
    3. Its ability to inactivate cholinesterase
    4. Its stimulant action on the motor nerve terminals at the motor end plate

10. _______ All of the following are associated with the effects of reserpine EXCEPT:

    1. Hypotenstion
    2. Parkinsonism-like syndrome
    3. Therapeutic in agitated schizophrenics
    4. Depletion of body stores of norepinephrine and serotonin
    5. Blockade of the peripheral effects of injected norepinephrine

<u>ONE BEST ANSWER</u>

11. _______ Each of the following impairs transmission at the neuromuscular junction EXCEPT:

    1. Diethyl ether
    2. Scopolamine
    3. Streptomycin
    4. Botulinus toxin
    5. d-Tubocurarine

12. _______ Competitive or non-depolarizing block at the neuromuscular junction is produced by all of the following EXCEPT:

    1. Decamethonium
    2. Gallamine
    3. Atracurium
    4. Curare

13. _______ Profound skeletal muscle paralysis develops in a patient after he is given a dose of tubocurarine which ordinarily does not produce detectable paralysis. What condition is this patient most likely to have?

    1. Myotonia congenita
    2. Myasthenia gravis
    3. Multiple sclerosis
    4. Atypical pseudocholinesterase
    5. None of the above

14. _______ Which one of the following drugs act <u>preferentially</u> to block pre-synaptic <u>alpha</u>-receptors on sympathetic nerve endings?

    1. Epinephrine
    2. Clonidine
    3. Phenylephrine
    4. Yohimbine
    5. Prazosin

15. _______ Low concentrations of sympathomimetic agents which are ineffective in the normal individual might produce a hypertensive response in a person treated chronically with which one of the following drugs?

    1. Tyramine
    2. Atropine
    3. Guanethidine
    4. Propranolol
    5. Phentolamine

<u>ONE BEST ANSWER</u>

16. _______ Tachycardia would most likely be observed following chronic administration of:

    1. Guanethidine
    2. Clonidine
    3. Reserpine
    4. Hydralazine
    5. Propranolol

17. _______ An anesthetized dog is pretreated with scopolamine and phentolamine. Intravenous administration of carbachol might be expected to produce a(n)
_______ in blood pressure:

    1. Increase
    2. Decrease
    3. No change

18. _______ In the above example the firing rate of the postganglionic nerves would _______ in response to carbachol:

    1. Increase
    2. Decrease
    3. Not change

<u>MULTIPLE TRUE-FALSE</u>
Directions: For each of the statements below, <u>ONE</u> or <u>MORE</u> of the completions given is correct.

    1 – If only 1, 2 and 3 are correct
    2 – If only 1 and 3 are correct
    3 – If only 2 and 4 are correct
    4 – If only 4 is correct
    5 – If all are correct

19. _______ Which of the following drugs will rapidly increase blood pressure in an animal pretreated chronically with reserpine?

    1. Phenylephrine
    2. Metaraminol
    3. Norepinephrine
    4. Tyramine

<u>MULTIPLE TRUE – FALSE</u>
<u>Directions Summarized:</u>

1	2	3	4	5
1,2,3	1,3	2,4	4	all are
only	only	only	only	correct

20. _______ Which of the following actions of propranolol might contribute to its hypotensive actions?

    1. Inhibition of central sympathetic tone
    2. Inhibition of renin release
    3. Decrease in cardiac output
    4. Blockade of peripheral <u>beta</u>-receptors on blood vessels

21. _______ Intravenous administration of norepinephrine produces a decrease in heart rate. Which of the following effects are causally related to this norepinephrine induced bradycardia:

    1. Increase in carotid sinus nerve activity
    2. Decrease in sympathetic nerve tone to heart
    3. Increase in efferent vagal nerve activity
    4. Stimulation of <u>beta</u>-adrenoreceptors in skeletal muscle vessels

22. _______ Administration of which of the following agents would prevent both the cardiac and vascular actions of intravenous tyramine injection:

    1. Atropine and phenoxybenzamine
    2. Reserpine
    3. Phenoxybenzamine and hexamethonium
    4. Phenoxybenzamine and propranolol

23. _______ A patient who has miosis, increased gut motility, excessive salivation and "spasm of accommodation" may have been given a therapeutic dose of which of the following drugs:

    1. Neostigmine
    2. Chlorisondamine
    3. Pilocarpine
    4. Phentolamine

24. _______ Side effects of <u>both</u> reserpine and guanethidine include:

    1. Bradycardia
    2. CNS depression
    3. Diarrhea
    4. Tachycardia

<u>MULTIPLE TRUE - FALSE</u>
Directions Summarized:

1	2	3	4	5
1,2,3	1,3	2,4	4	all are
only	only	only	only	correct

25. _______ Drugs that lower blood pressure by a direct action on vascular smooth
muscle may cause, by a reflex mechanism, which of the following?

    1. Bradycardia
    2. Release of renin
    3. Cycloplegia
    4. Increased sympathetic nerve activity

26. _______ Which of the following agents might potentiate the degree of
neuromuscular blockade produced by d-tubocurarine?

    1. Streptomycin
    2. Neostigmine
    3. Ether
    4. Epinephrine

27. _______ Which of the following agents act primarily by a presynaptic
mechanism to alter cholinergic function?

    1. Hemicholinium
    2. Tetrodotoxin
    3. Botulinus toxin
    4. Snake <u>alpha</u>-toxins

28. _______ Dobutamine:

    1. Produces dilation of renal blood vessels
    2. Is effective orally
    3. Is refractory to inactivation by MAO
    4. Is useful primarily because of its stimulation of B_1 receptors

29. _______ Epinephrine:

    1. Increases the contractile force of the heart
    2. Increases the automaticity of the heart
    3. Causes local vasoconstriction if injected subcutaneously
    4. Dilates arterioles in skeletal muscles.

30. _______ Side effects of hexamethonium administration include:

    1. Diarrhea
    2. Cycloplegia
    3. Excessive sweating
    4. Postural hypotension

<u>MULTIPLE TRUE – FALSE</u>
<u>Directions Summarized:</u>

1	2	3	4	5
1,2,3	1,3	2,4	4	all are
only	only	only	only	correct

31. _______ Which drug(s) form enzyme-substrate complexes with cholinesterases of longer duration than that formed with acetylcholine?

1. Physostigmine
2. Pilocarpine
3. Diisopropylfluorophosphate (DFP)
4. Atropine

32. _______ Isoproterenol:

1. Increases the automaticity of the sinoatrial (SA) node
2. Effectively increases ventricular rate in the presence of complete A-V heart block (Stoke-Adams syndrome)
3. Relaxes bronchiolar smooth muscle in the presence of bronchial asthma
4. Reduces peripheral resistance

33. _______ Succinylcholine acts by:

1. Inhibiting acetylcholine release
2. Depolarizing nerve terminals
3. Blocking acetylcholine receptors
4. Depolarizing muscle end plate receptors

34. _______ d-Tubocurarine:

1. Blocks the effect of acetylcholine on muscle end plate receptors
2. Prevents the release of acetylcholine from the motor nerve terminals
3. Enhances the curariform action of ether
4. Causes transient fasciculations before paralysis develops

35. _______ Phentolamine:

1. Increases arterial blood pressure.
2. Increases heart rate reflexly
3. Decreases myocardial contractile force
4. Is used for the diagnosis of pheochromocytoma

36. _______ <u>Beta</u> adrenergic blocking drugs such as propranolol can block:

1. The increase in cardiac contractile force and heart rate caused by sympathetic nerve stimulation
2. The vasodilator response to isoproterenol
3. The bronchodilator action of epinephrine
4. The bronchodilator action of theophylline

<u>MULTIPLE TRUE - FALSE</u>
<u>Directions Summarized:</u>

1	2	3	4	5
1,2,3	1,3	2,4	4	all are
only	only	only	only	correct

37. _______ Hexamethonium:

1. Is poorly and variably absorbed from the gastrointestinal tract after oral administration
2. Does not readily cross the blood brain barrier
3. Can prevent acetylcholine, released from autonomic preganglionic fibers, from acting on autonomic postganglionic cell bodies
4. Can cause a dry mouth

38. _______ Stimulation of the splanchnic nerves might be expected to release which of the following substances into the circulation?

1. ATP
2. Norepinephrine
3. Dopamine <u>beta</u>-hydroxylase
4. Epinephrine

39. _______ Which of the following metabolic effects would be expected in response to an injection of epinephrine?

1. Decrease of hepatic glycogen
2. Increase of hepatic phosphorylase <u>a</u>
3. Decrease of glycogen synthetase <u>a</u>
4. Increased lipogenesis in adipose tissue

40. _______ Metaproterenol:

1. Is a selective B_1 agonist
2. Relaxes uterine smooth muscle
3. Is a selective B_1 antagonist
4. Is useful in treatment of asthma

41. _______ Treatment of organophosphorus insecticide poisoning might rationally require the prompt administration of:

1. Morphine
2. Atropine
3. Phenobarbital
4. Pralidoxime (2-PAM)

42. _______ Which of the following neuromuscular blocking agents might be used in patients with severe renal disease?

1. Gallamine
2. Atricurium
3. Pancuronium
4. Succinylcholine

<u>MULTIPLE TRUE - FALSE</u>
<u>Directions Summarized:</u>

1	2	3	4	5
1,2,3	1,3	2,4	4	all are
only	only	only	only	correct

43. _______ Imipramine would be expected to inhibit the actions of which of the
following drugs?

    1.   Tyramine
    2.   6-OH dopamine
    3.   Guanethidine
    4.   Amphetamine

44. _______ Which of the following agents bind tightly <u>only</u> to the esteratic site
of acetylcholinesterase?

    1.   Parathion
    2.   Physostigmine
    3.   Isofluorophate
    4.   Edrophonium

<u>MATCHING</u>

Choose the one most appropriate response – use each choice only once

1. Chlorisondamine
2. Reserpine
3. <u>Alpha</u> methyl para tyrosine
4. Hydralazine
5. Methyldopa

6. 6-Hydroxydopamine
7. Chlorthalidone
8. Phentolamine
9. Guanethidine
10. Pargyline

45. _______ Diuretic antihypertensive drug

46. _______ Potential false transmitter precursor

47. _______ Chronic treatment depletes CNS monoamines

48. _______ Has actions similar to both reserpine and bretylium

49. _______ Orally effective ganglionic blocker

50. _______ Direct vasodilator of vascular smooth muscle

51. _______ Inhibits MAO

52. _______ Blocks <u>alpha</u> receptors by competitive action

53. _______ Inhibits tyrosine hydroxylase

54. _______ Selectively destructive to adrenergic nerve endings
Choose the one most appropriate response – use each choice only once

* * * * * * * * *

1. Metoprolol
2. Methamphetamine
3. Methoxamine
4. Metanephrine
5. Metaproterenol

55. _______ Metabolite formed by action of COMT on epinephrine

56. _______ Stimulates <u>alpha</u> receptors directly

57. _______ An "indirect" acting sympathomimetic

58. _______ "Cardioselective" adrenergic blocking drug

59. _______ "Selective" <u>beta</u>$_2$ stimulant (agonist)

<u>MATCHING</u>

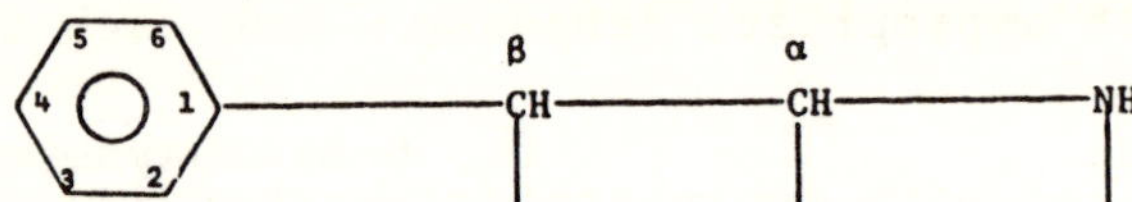

1. Hydroxy groups on positions 3 and 4 of ring
2. Methyl substitution on α-carbon
3. Hydroxy substitution on β-carbon
4. Hydroxy groups on positions 3 and 5 of ring
5. Dextrorotatory substitution on nitrogen

Match the above alterations or substitution of the phenylethylamine core structure that will most likely produce the following alterations of action of sympathetic drugs.

60. _______ Resistant to COMT; increased β_2 receptor selectivity

61. _______ Must be present for uptake and storage in neuronal storage granules

62. _______ Protects amine from inactivation by MAO

* * * * * * * * * *

1. Dobutamine
2. Ritodrine
3. Both
4. Neither

63. _______ "Selective" beta adrenoceptor agonist

64. _______ Orally effective

65. _______ Antagonizes cardiac actions of norepinephrine

<u>MATCHING</u>

A number may be used more than once.

In a dog anesthetized with pentobarbital, recording electrodes are placed on:

I   Carotid sinus baroreceptor nerve fibers
II Splanchnic (sympathetic) nerve fibers (preganglionic)
III Inferior cardiac (sympathetic) nerve fibers (postganglionic)
IV Vagal (parasympathetic) nerve fibers

What changes (if any) in firing rates would be expected to occur following the administration of the <u>last</u> drug in each series of drugs listed below? Presume that sufficient time for the actions of the premedicating agents has been allowed and then the last agent is given intravenously.

Give one answer for each set of nerves (in order I-IV) from the choices below. ↑ = increase of nerve activity; ↓ = decrease nerve activity; ↔ = no change in neural firing.

	I	II	III	IV
1.	↔	↔	↔	↔
2.	↑	↓	↓	↑
3.	↔	↓	↓	↑
4.	↓	↑	↑	↓
5.	↑	↓	↔	↑

66. _______ Propranolol, and atropine; then <u>phenylephrine</u>

67. _______ Propranolol, atropine and reserpine; then <u>phenylephrine</u>

68. _______ Propranolol, atropine, reserpine and hexamethonium; then <u>phenylephrine</u>

69. _______ Propranolol, atropine, reserpine, hexamethonium and phenoxybenzamine; then <u>phenylephrine</u>

70. _______ What changes (if any) would be expected in the firing rates in the above four nerves following <u>bilateral common carotid artery occlusion</u> in an animal that had been pretreated with atropine, phentolamine and propranolol

<u>MATCHING</u>

The following tracings represent the changes in mean systemic blood pressure
in an anesthetized dog in response to drugs A, B, C and D given intravenously.
The first panel shows the control responses, the second panel shows the
responses after reserpine pretreatment. The last panel shows the responses
after <u>subsequent</u> administration of atropine. The same dose of each agent is
given in each case.

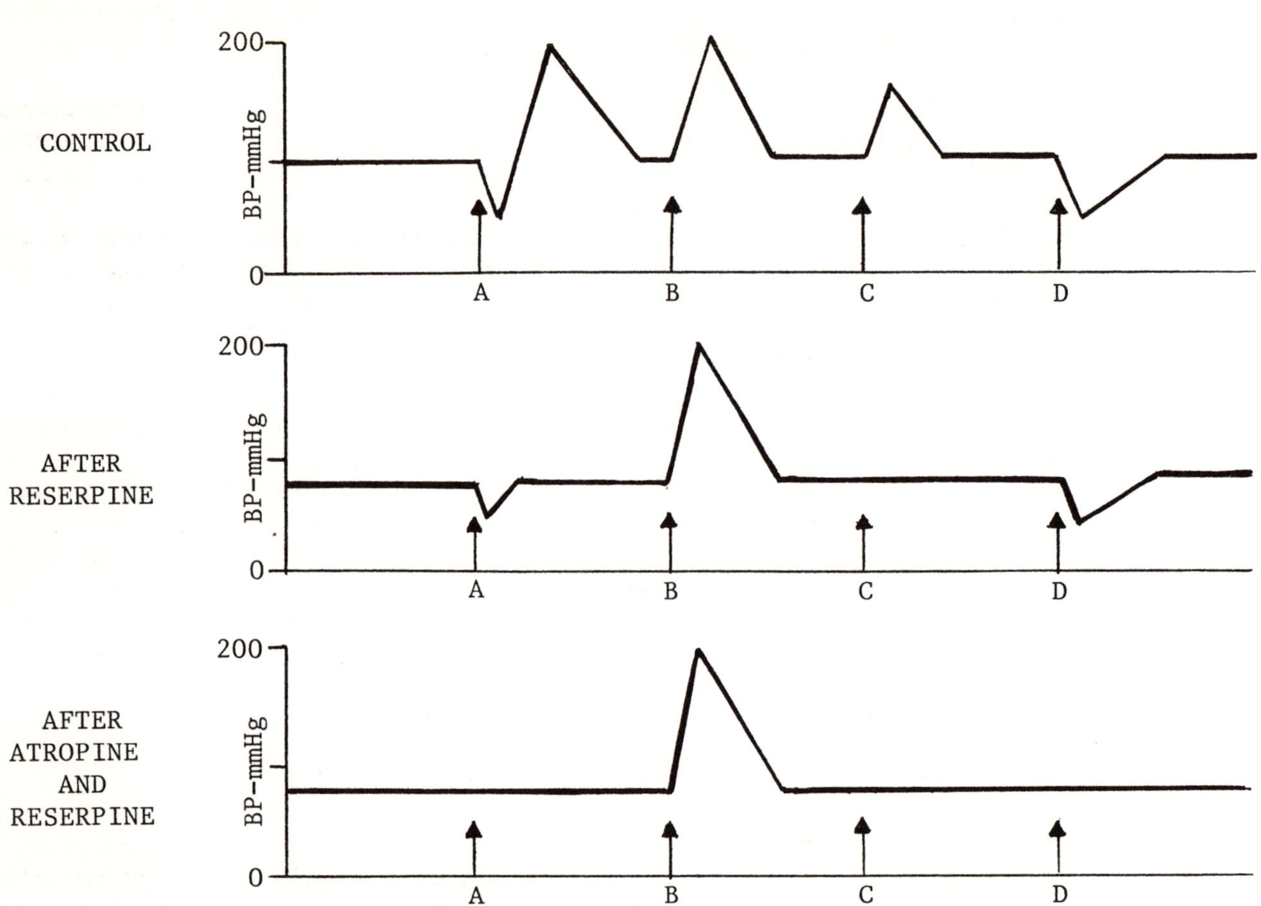

From the above information what are drugs A - D?

71. _______ Drug A is:

    1. Nicotine
    2. Hexamethonium
    3. Trimethaphan
    4. Ephedrine
    5. Norepinephrine

73. _______ Drug C is:

    1. Norepinephrine
    2. Tyramine
    3. Epinephrine
    4. Phenylephrine
    5. Isoproterenol

72. _______ Drug B is:

    1. Nicotine
    2. Histamine
    3. Ephedrine
    4. Isoproterenol
    5. Phenylephrine

74. _______ Drug D is:

    1. Tyramine
    2. Ephedrine
    3. Pilocarpine
    4. Phenylephrine
    5. Histamine

<u>MATCHING</u>

The following bar graphs represent changes in blood pressure measured in an anesthetized dog. (+) equals an increase and (–) equals a decrease in blood pressure in response to intravenous administration of drugs A–D. The first series of responses are controls (no pretreatment). The second, third, fourth and fifth series are responses to the <u>same</u> drugs following pretreatment of the agents P–S administered sequentially. Regard the effect of the pretreatment as being complete and lasting throughout the experiment. Identify unknown drugs A–D and each pretreatment or blocker P–S.

<u>Drugs (A–D)</u>

1. Acetylcholine (100 μg/kg)
2. Methacholine
3. Tyramine
4. Norepinephrine
5. Angiotensin

<u>Pretreatment (P–S)</u>

1. Atropine
2. Reserpine
3. Phenoxybenzamine
4. Hexamethonium
5. Propranolol

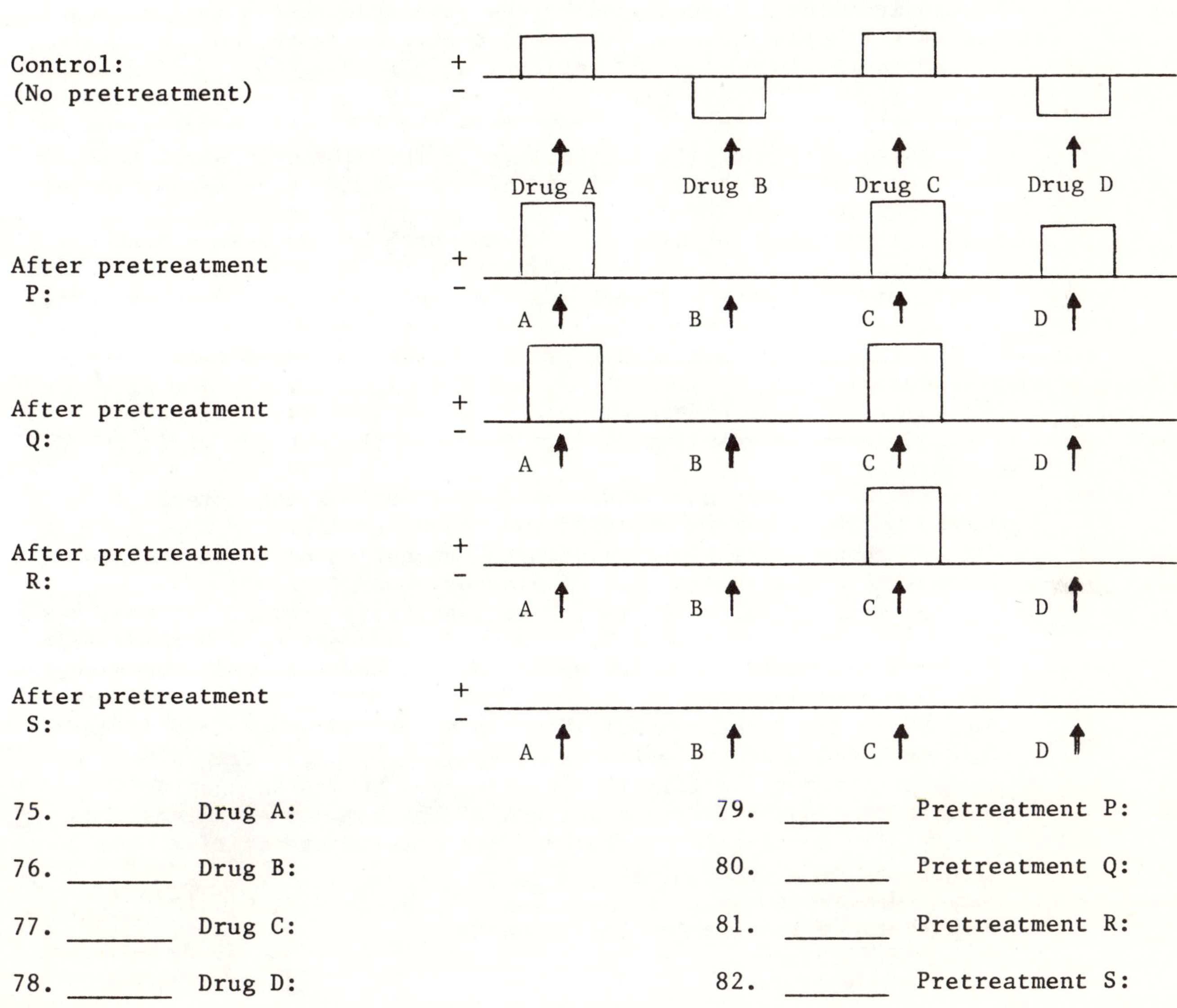

75. _______ Drug A:

76. _______ Drug B:

77. _______ Drug C:

78. _______ Drug D:

79. _______ Pretreatment P:

80. _______ Pretreatment Q:

81. _______ Pretreatment R:

82. _______ Pretreatment S:

ANSWERS

1.   5   The sequence of NE synthesis is: phenylalanine → tyrosine → DOPA dopamine → NE. VMA is the major metabolite found in the urine after both COMT and MAO have degraded NE.

2.   4   Contraction of the radial muscle of the iris results in mydriasis. This is mediated via alpha adrenergic receptors, i.e., blocked by phenoxybenzamine and phentolamine but not by propranolol.

3.   3   Atropine administration causes mydriasis or dilation of the pupil in that the predominant parasympathetic tone is blocked. This might precipitate or worsen glaucoma. Atropine would have little if any effect in the other conditions mentioned.

4.   3   All of the mentioned compounds except for carbachol would be effective in asthma by directly or indirectly relaxing bronchial smooth muscle. If any thing, carbachol might cause further contraction.

5.   1

6.   5   Theophylline relaxes bronchial smooth muscle and is useful in treating asthma.

7.   3   Succinylcholine is hydrolyzed by the same type of enzyme that breaks down ACh (cholinesterase). Choline acetylase is the enzyme involved in the synthesis of ACh and anticholinesterase agents complex with cholinesterase thus increasing the time ACh can exert its actions.

8.   4   Remember that the adrenergic receptors that NE acts on are alpha in the vasculature and beta in the heart. Thus the only agent that would produce the above metnioned effects would be an alpha blocker, i.e., phenoxybenzamine.

9.   3   Neostigmine complexes with the enzyme which breaks down ACh thus increases its effectiveness and duration at the NMJ. Remember that neostigmine also has a direct stimulation action on the postsynaptic receptors. Thus it has a dual effect, and consequently, is a drug of choice in treating myasthenia gravis. Motor nerve terminals are pre-synaptic.

10.   5   Reserpine depletes endogenous norepinephrine stores. Depletion of the endogenous transmitter will not reduce the actions of injected norepinephrine.

11.   2   Scopolamine acts at muscarinic receptors but has no appreciable effect on the nicotinic type of receptors found at the NMJ.

12.   1   All are competitive blockers with the exception of decamethonium which is a depolarizing type of blocker.

13.   2   This patient is most likely to have myasthenia gravis. If he already has a deficit in neuromuscular function, a competitive blocker like tubocurarine would be effective at lower doses than would be expected in the normal individual.

14.   4   Yohimbine acts "preferentially" as an $alpha_2$ adrenoceptor blocker (the type found at pre-synaptic peripheral sites). Clonidine also has a preference for this type of receptor but as an agonist.

15.   3   Guanethidine would decrease release of NE from nerve endings thus potentially causing the receptors to become supersensitive to a direct acting sympathomimetic drug.

16.   4   Only hydralazine would decrease blood pressure without also reducing sympathetic effectiveness to the heart.

17.   2   Carbachol would stimulate autonomic ganglia and the adrenal gland. Since both the non-innervated muscaric receptors and the innervated <u>alpha</u> receptors on blood vessels are blocked, the circulating epinephrine from the adrenal gland would act on the non-innervated <u>beta</u> receptors to produce vasodilation and a lowering of blood pressure.

18.   1   The nerve activity would increase due to both the direct ganglionic action of carbachol as well as the reflex compensation due to decreased blood pressure.

19.   1   Reserpine treatment will deplete nerve terminal of NE, but direct acting agents will still have effect (potentially exaggerated due to supersensitivity). Tyramine is indirect and will act only if NE is in nerve terminal to be released.

20.   1   Blockade of <u>beta</u>-receptors will not affect blood pressure as these receptors are not tonically activated and, even if so, would produce opposite effect.

21.   1   The reflex response to direct <u>alpha</u> activated increase in pressure would involve afferents as well as sympathetic and parasympathetic efferents (to heart). NE does not act potently on vascular <u>beta</u>-receptors.

22.   3   Reserpine would deplete the catecholamine stores in nerve endings, thus preventing the actions of the indirect-acting sympathomimetic. PBZ and propranolol would block the <u>alpha</u> and <u>beta</u> actions of released NE.

23.   2   Both the anticholinesterase agent, neostigmine, and direct muscarinic agonist, pilocarpine, would produce these parasympathomimetic effects.

24.   2   Guanethidine does not get into CNS thus causes no CNS depression. Neither agent would produce elevated heart rate.

25.   3   The reflex response would be to increase sympathetic and decrease vagal tone. Renin is released by sympathetic nerves to kidney.

26.   2   Neostigmine and epinephrine would antagonize the blockade of a competitive NMJ blocker by increasing the amount of ACh in the synapse by enzyme inhibition and Ca^{++} mediated facilitation of release respectively.

27.   1   Snake <u>alpha</u>-toxins act postsynaptically by binding with the nicotinic ACh receptor.

28.   4   Only answer four is correct. Don't confuse the name with dopamine.

29.   5   Epinephrine acts strongly on both <u>alpha</u> and <u>beta</u> adrenergic receptors throughout the body. Thus all of the effects listed would be expected to occur.

30.   3   Ganglionic blockade would cause constipation and lack of sweating. Cycloplegia (paralysis of accomodation) occurs as parasympathetic tone is necessary for near vision. Postural hypotension is a result of both decreased sympathetic tone and lack of reflex compensation after ganglion block.

31.   2   Both physostigmine and DFP are effective anticholinesterase agents for the reason mentioned in this question. Pilocarpine and atropine act only on the muscarinic receptor as a stimulant and blocker respectively.

32.   5   All are correct. Isoproterenol acts directly on the <u>beta</u> adrenergic receptors in the heart to increase both rate and force of contraction. In addition, it acts on the <u>beta</u> receptors in bronchiolar and vascular smooth muscle causing relaxation of these muscles.

33.   4   Succinylcholine acts on the <u>postsynaptic</u> receptor as a depolarizing neuromuscular blocking agent. It does not act at the presynaptic element.

34.   2   This agent acts postsynaptically as a competitive type of neuromuscular blocking agent and is synergistic with the similar effects of ether. Succinylcholine, but not d-tubocurarine, causes transient fasciculations prior to paralysis.

35.   3   Phentolamine is a short acting competitive blocker of <u>alpha</u> adrenergic receptors. Thus it will lower blood pressure (reduction of sympathetic tone effectiveness) and cause a reflex increase in heart rate. It has no <u>direct</u> action in the heart <u>(beta</u> receptors) and is used to diagnosis phenochromocytoma.

36.   1   Propranolol blocks the peripheral and cardiac <u>beta</u> receptors. It will not block the non-<u>beta</u> receptor mediated action of theophylline.

37.   5 C_6 has a N^+ group therefore is not readily absorbed nor can it readily cross the B.B.B. It, like other ganglionic blockers acts on the postsynaptic nicotinic ganglion receptors and one of the results of this is dry mouth (xerostomia).

38.   5   Activation of the splanchnic nerves releases Epi and NE from the adrenal medulla. The ATP and enzyme are also in storage granules and will be released with the catecholamines.

39.   1

40.   3

41.   3   Atropine will relieve the peripheral and CNS over-activation of muscarinic mechanisms, thus offering some relief. 2-PAM is an enzyme reactivator and is effective for many types of organophosphorous agents.

42.   3

43.   1

44.   2

45.   7

46.   5

47.   2

48.   9

49.   1

50.   4

51.   10

52.   8

53.   3

54.   6

55.   4

56.   3

57.   2

58.   1

59.   5

60.   4   Hydroxy substitution at 3 and 5 is characteristic of orally effective <u>beta</u>-2-agonists. See page II-35.

61.   3   Hydroxylation of <u>beta</u> carbon is needed for transport into storage granules.

62.   2   A methyl substitution on the <u>alpha</u> carbon makes the molecule resistant to attack by MAO which acts at the terminal nitrogen.

63.   3

64.   2

65.   4

66. – 70.   Phenylephrine will cause an elevation of blood pressure due to direct
alpha-adrenoceptor stimulation. The response in these nerves to
increased pressure is to increase firing in the carotid sinus
afferent nerves which excites vagal outflow and inhibits the
sympathetic efferent outflow to the blood vessels and heart as in
question #66. In question #67 the answer will be the same because
depletion of NE by reserpine would only augment the pressor action of
phenylephrine. In #68 hexamethonium (C_6) will block efferent
ganglionic transmission, thus no activity is possible in the
post-ganglionic nerves. In #69, phenoxybenzamine will prevent the
pressor effect of phenylephrine, thus no change in blood pressure and
no change in firing of nerves. The final question (#70) demonstrates
that the neural response to carotid occlusion still occurs even
though the blood pressure does not change due to blockade of all
relevant end organs.

66.   2
67.   2
68.   5
69.   1
70.   4

71.   1   When nicotine is given i.v. the first organ to see the drug is the
heart where parasympathetic ganglia are located in the muscle wall.
Then as the nicotine is pumped around it can then activate the
sympathetic ganglia and adrenal gland. This provides the biphasic
response shown. Reserpine eliminates the pressor response; atropine
blocks the depressor response due to severe slowing of heart rate.

72.   5   Drug B must be a direct acting sympathomimetic (alpha) as effect is
potentiated by amine depletion. Ephedrine would be partially reduced
in effect by depletion as about half of its actions are indirect
(release of NE from nerve endings).

73.   2   Drug C must be an indirect acting sympathomimetic as the action is
blocked by depletion of NE with reserpine.

74.   3   Drug D is blocked by atropine. Thus pilocarpine acts on
non-innervated muscarinic receptors of vasculature causing
vasodilation.

75. – 82.   First look at over-all problem and note that all effects are
eventually blocked. As there is no angiotensin receptor blocker in
the pretreatment group you can discard angiotensin as a potential
answer. Pressor drugs (A and C) could be either tyramine or
norepinephrine (NE). Depressor drugs are either acetylcholine (ACh)
or methacholine. As drug B is blocked and the large dose of ACh
shows reversal of action (depressor to pressor) the only possible
answer is drug B = methacholine and drug D = ACh and blocker P =
atropine. The reversal of ACh after atropine is a ganglionic
stimulating effect, thus pretreatment Q must be the ganglionic
blocker hexamethonium. With regard to the two pressor drugs,
depletion of the endogenous stores of NE would selectively prevent
the actions of the indirect sympathomimetic, tyramine. Alpha
receptor blockade would block both NE and tyramine. Thus agonist A
is tyramine and R is reserpine. Agonist C is NE which is blocked by
pretreatment S, phenoxybenzamine.

75.   3   79.   1
76.   2   80.   4
77.   4   81.   2
78.   1   82.   3

SECTION III: <u>CENTRAL NERVOUS SYSTEM DRUGS</u>

GENERAL ANESTHETICS

General anesthetics are central nervous system depressants used in surgery to produce loss of sensation to pain (analgesia) and loss of consciousness; ideally the anesthetic agents also should provide good muscle relaxation and reduction of reflex activity. Medullary areas controlling respiration and the cardiovascular system are spared with low concentrations of anesthetics but are progressively depressed when larger concentrations are administered.

I. Stages of Anesthesia: well defined signs of anesthesia were described by Guedel using open-drop ether anesthesia with no preanesthetic medication. These stages may not be applicable to other anesthetic agents.

Stage I   – <u>Analgesia</u>: Amnesia is also common during this stage.

Stage II – <u>Delirium or Excitement</u>: Begins with unconsciousness; involuntary movement and struggling; irregular respiration; dilated pupils; vomiting; excitement.

Stage III – <u>Surgical Anesthesia</u>: Divided into 4 planes; based on progressive respiratory depression, muscular relaxation and loss of reflexes.

Stage IV – <u>Medullary Paralysis</u>:

II. Inhalation Anesthetics:

   A. <u>Gaseous</u> – <u>Nitrous oxide</u>: Incomplete anesthetic (>100 MAC), CNS-analgesia, increase in cerebral blood flow and intracranial pressure, dose related sensory changes. Reproduction – slight increase in spontaneous abortions. "Recreational" misuse–neuropathy with distal numbness, weakness, incoordination and amnesia.

   B. <u>Volatile Liquids</u> – <u>Halothane</u>, <u>Enflurane</u> and <u>Isoflurane</u>: No specific analgesic action; cerebral vasodilation, hypotension; relaxation of uterine smooth muscle; reduction in renal blood flow, glomerular filtration rate and urinary flow rate; potential for malignant hyperthermia. <u>Major differences</u> – Halothane has the greatest potential for ventricular arrhythmia with circulating catecholamine; Halothane may cause bradycardia, tachypnea and hepatitis; Enflurane may cause tonic-clonic seizures with hypocapnea.

   C. Factors affecting inhalation anesthesia
      1. partial pressure of anesthetic in inspired gas (concentration)
      2. the rate of uptake of anesthetic by the blood (blood/gas partition coefficient or blood solubility)
      3. the rate of uptake of anesthetic by the tissues (blood flow and tissue/blood partition coefficient or tissue solubility)
      4. speed of induction (and emergence) is inversely correlated with the blood/gas partition coefficient
      5. agents with high blood solubility (partition coefficient for ether 12.1, halothane 2.3) induce anesthesia more slowly than agents that are poorly soluble in blood (partition coefficient for nitrous oxide 0.47); when an agent is highly soluble in blood, more of the agent has to be dissolved in blood before an adequate concentration can be achieved in the brain; this causes induction to be slow.
      6. relative potencies of inhalation anesthetics are determined by the minimal alveolar concentration (MAC) that will produce anesthesia in 50% of patients to a noxious stimulus (response to skin incision); this is an ED_{50}.

III. Intravenous Anesthetics:
    A. <u>Induction Agents</u>
       1. <u>Ultra-short acting barbiturates</u>: thiopental, methohexital:
          Induction rapid and pleasant; poor analgesia; laryngospasm; poor
          muscle relaxation; dose-related cardiovascular depression; no liver
          toxicity; repeated doses result in prolonged recovery, as drug will
          redistribute and accumulate in body tissues.
       2. <u>Etomidate</u>: Non-barbiturate hypnotic without analgesic properties
          that has less cardiovascular and respiratory depressant actions than
          thiopental; hydrolyzed by liver and plasma esterases.
       3. <u>Midazolam</u>: Water-soluble benzodiazepine.
    B. <u>Sedative Agents Used i.v. For Outpatient Surgery</u> (Conscious Sedation)
       1. <u>Diazepam</u>, <u>Lorazepam</u> or <u>Midazolam</u> i.v. are the primarily agents; for
          analgesic effects, the high potency narcotic <u>Fentanyl</u> is used.
          Other narcotics have been used (e.g. pentazocine) but they do not
          offer an advantage over fentanyl and may be more dangerous. If an
          anesthetic supplement is required, <u>methohexital</u> should be used in
          place of diazepam.
    C. <u>Oral and Intramuscular Sedative Agents</u>
       1. <u>Chloral hydrate</u> with <u>hydroxyzine</u>: Used in children (see
          sedative-hypnotic section).
       2. <u>Ketamine</u>: Dissociative anesthetic; structurally related to
          phenylcyclidine (PCP); good analgesia and amnesia; awakening is
          prolonged; disagreeable dreams and hallucinations; used in burn
          centers, for head and neck operations and in high risk patients.

IV. <u>Balanced Anesthesia</u>
    Combination of agents used to facilitate induction and maintenance of
anesthesia, as no one anesthetic agent has all the desirable properties
required for surgical anesthesia; advantages are that small concentrations
of anesthetic are needed and less cardiovascular depression occurs.
    1. <u>Preanesthetic Medication</u>: Used to facilitate induction and maintenance
       of anesthesia. Sedative-hypnotic: given to allay anxiety and/or promote
       sleep the night before and again before anesthesia. Narcotic: to
       alleviate pre- and post-operative pain. Anticholinergic: to minimize
       problems of excessive secretions and reflex bradycardia.
    2. <u>Induction</u>: Ultrashort acting barbiturate
    3. <u>Neuromuscular blocking agent</u>: Succinylcholine or curare to provide
       adequate muscular relaxation (effects of curare are potentiated by
       ether, halothane, enflurane and methoxyflurane)
    4. <u>Anesthetic</u>: Nitrous oxide is used as the carrier gas; this speeds the
       uptake and distribution of the second inhalation agent and also reduces
       the concentration needed of the second agent.

LOCAL ANESTHETICS

Local anesthetics: Reversibly block conduction along the axon

Ester type	Amide type
Procaine	Lidocaine
Chlorprocaine	Prilocaine
Tetracaine	Dibucaine
Cocaine	Mepivacaine
	Bupivacaine
	Etidocaine

a. Most are weak bases; penetrate as unionized form into neuron where they reequilibrate to both charged and uncharged forms; inside the neuron, the positively charged ion blocks nerve conduction by preventing inward flow of sodium ions and propagation of action potential.

b. The absorption depends upon the vascularity and blood flow to the area. Often given with epinephrine or other vasoconstrictor to prolong anesthesia. With application to pharynx or respiratory tract you can get very high blood levels. Metabolism: ester types hydrolysed by esterases in plasma, while the amide types are metabolized in the liver.

c. Hypersensitivity can occur (several texts suggest it is quite rare): manifestations include rashes, asthma and anaphylaxis – more frequent with ester linkage type.

d. Overdose toxicity – May get initial CNS stimulation (ranging from anxiety, tremors to convulsions), later depression to areflexia, coma, extreme hypotension and respiratory failure.

e. Procaine – prototype ester: anesthesia 1 hr.

Lidocaine – prototype amide: most widely used of any local anesthetic, intermediate duration (1–3 hr), sleepiness is a common side effect.

Tetracaine, dibucaine, bupivacaine, and etidocaine are long acting (3–8 hr).

Prilocaine can produce methemoglobinemia.

Cocaine: produces vasoconstriction, limited use for topical application to mucosa of nose and pharynx.

SEDATIVE – HYPNOTICS

Certain general depressants of the CNS are used to relieve anxiety, to sedate or to induce sleep (hypnosis). The magnitude of their effects is dose-dependent. Besides their sedative, hypnotic and anxiolytic properties as a class they are characterized by being anticonvulsants, CNS muscle relaxants, anesthetics and their ability to develop physical dependence.

I. <u>BARBITURATES</u>

1. Mechanism of action is primarily by a receptor site at or near the chloride ionophore of the benzodiazepine-GABA receptor ($GABA_A$ receptor) complex. Secondarily they may inhibit adenosine uptake. Lipid solubility affects the onset and duration of response. The two most important substitutions are sulfur (thio) at C_2 to increase the lipid solubility for use as i.v. anesthetics (<u>thiopental</u>) and phenyl at C_5 (<u>phenobarbital</u>) which results in anticonvulsant activity at subhypnotic doses.

2. Termination of action: physical redistribution (single dose, ultra short acting barbiturates-<u>thiopental</u>, <u>methohexital</u>); metabolism-generally to hydroxyl compound (most barbiturates-<u>pentobarbital</u>, <u>secobarbital</u>), and excretion (long acting barbiturates-<u>phenobarbital</u>).

3. Induce cytochrome P-450 microsomal enzyme activity which increases rate of their own metabolism and also other drugs metabolized by this system; also induces aminolevulinic synthetase, the rate limiting step in heme biosynthesis, and thus are contraindicated in patients with acute intermittent porphyria, porphyria variegata or a positive family history of these porphyrias.

4. Tolerance to sedative and hypnotic effects and true physical dependence develops. Tolerance due to both CNS cellular adapation and microsomal enzyme induction. No tolerance develops to lethal dose or to anticonvulsant property.

5. Withdrawal characteristics: anxiety, stomach cramps, nausea and vomiting, orthostatic hypotension, and mild tremor start 12-16 hours after the last dose of a short-acting barbiturate. Peak occurs at 2-3 days with tonic-clonic type convulsions, and if the patient survives, toxic psychosis, exhaustion and cardiovascular collapse are a problem. After about a week the withdrawal symptoms subside. Taking doses of 800 mg/day of pentobarbital or secobarbital for several weeks followed by abrupt withdrawal will cause 75% of patients to have at least one convulsion and 60% toxic psychosis. The toxic psychosis is not easily reversed once it begins. Deaths do occur during barbiturate withdrawal.

6. Acute poisoning: most important treatment is supportive, maintain airway, assist ventilation if necessary. Hemodialysis and alkalinization of urine helpful only with long acting barbiturates.

7. Contraindications and cautions:
   Acute intermittent porphyria
   Allergic reactions
   Hepatic or renal disease
   Drug interactions related to induction of liver microsomal enzymes.

II. <u>BENZODIAZEPINES</u>

1. Marketing rather than pharmacological profile is the prime determinant
   in classification of the benzodiazepines. Hypnotics: <u>Flurazepam</u>,
   temazepam, <u>triazolam</u>, nitrazepam. Anxiolytics: <u>Diazepam</u>,
   chlordiazepoxide, oxazepam, <u>lorazepam</u>, <u>alprazolam</u>, chlorazepate,
   Anticonvulsant: clonazepam. Anesthetic Induction Agent: midazolam.

2. Mechanism of action: $GABA_A$ receptor, i.e., benzodiazepine-GABA receptor
   chloride ionophore complex.

3. No evidence that one benzodiazepine is clinically superior to another.
   Many have a common intermediate-nordiazepam or the halogenated
   nordiazepam, which have a 50–120 hour half-life.

4. Very limited evidence that any benzodiazepine is effective beyond four
   months of continuous use.

5. Some benzodiazepines, oxazepam, lorazepam and triazolam, alprazolam and
   midazolam have shorter half lifes so their potential to accumulate is
   less.

6. Anticonvulsant activity is enhanced in compounds having a nitro group
   (nitrazepam and clonazepam). Tolerance develops rapidly.

7. Compared to barbiturates and meprobamate, they are less likely to
   produce serious poisoning on overdose. Their abuse liability is also
   less. Physical dependence can occur, withdrawal symptoms are similar to
   those of the barbiturates.

8. Microsomal enzyme induction does not occur, but they can induce ALA
   synthetase.

III. <u>OTHER AGENTS</u>

1. <u>Buspirone</u>: Clinical efficacy for treatment of anxiety without other
   benzodiazepine properties, i.e., does <u>NOT</u> produce muscle relaxation,
   control seizures, produce sedation-hypnosis or physical dependence.

2. <u>Hydroxyzine</u>: Sedative-anxiolytic with antiemetic and slight
   atropine-like action.

3. <u>Chloral hydrate</u>: Metabolized to trichloroethanol; like barbiturates can
   induce drug metabolizing enzymes; contraindicated in patients with acute
   intermittent porphyria.

4. <u>Paraldehyde</u>: Polymer of aldehyde; offensive odor and disagreeable
   taste; significant amount of drug excreted unchanged through the lungs;
   could be used in some cases of hepatic or renal insufficiency.

5. <u>Methaqualone</u>: Can be used in patients with porphyria; peripheral neuropathy can occur, high doses may cause frank convulsions; dissociative high; widely abused. Removed from U.S. market.

6. Most over-the-counter sleep aids contain antihistamines and/or scopolamine.

7. Alcohol is the most widely used sedative-hypnotic.

IV. <u>TREATMENT: DRUGS OF CHOICE FOR ANXIETY STATES AND RELATED CONDITIONS</u>

1.	Situational anxiety	Benzodiazepines
2.	Anxiety with depression	Alprazolam most prescribed – not conclusive that it has a selective property.
3.	Obsessive-compulsions, panic disorders	Benzodiazepines Imipramine-clomipramine
4.	Phobias with or without agoraphobia (panic attacks)	Imipramine (lower dose than for treatment of depression) MAOI's-phenelzine
5.	Stage fright	Propranolol
6.	Parasomnias	
	a. Sleep walking	Diazepam
	b. Night terrors	Diazepam
	c. Sleep walkers with complex and at times violent behavior (atypical anterior-medial temporal lobe epilepsy)	Phenytoin or Carbamazepine
	d. Primary enuresis	Imipramine
	e. Sleep-related bruxism	Imipramine
7.	Narcolepsy	Amphetamine Methylphenidate
	a. Cataplexy	Imipramine

<u>ALCOHOLS</u>

Alcohols belong to the sedative-hypnotic CNS depressant class of drugs.

I. <u>Acute Ethanol Intoxication</u>

   A. Pharmacological Effects:

      1. <u>CNS Effects</u>: Depend on the blood alcohol concentration (BAC).

BAC %	Characteristics
0.015 – 0.055	Blurred Vision
0.05	"Legally Impaired"*
0.05 – 0.075	Delightful Dizziness, Muscular Incoordination Begins
0.075 – 0.100	Delayed Reaction Time
0.100	"Legally Intoxicated"*
0.150 – 0.200	Emotional Instability
0.200 – 0.300	Confusion, Slurred Speech
0.300 – 0.400	Stupor
0.400 – 0.500	Dead Drunk, Coma
0.500 – 0.600	Dead

         (*Legal limits for BAC vary with local governmental regulations)

      2. <u>Gastrointestinal</u>: Increased saliva and gastric secretions. Direct irritation to gastric and buccal mucosa, emesis due to central effect on chemoreceptor trigger zone and irritiation of gastric mucosa. Decreased absorption of folates.

      3. <u>Cardiovascular system</u>: Initial transient tachycardia and hypertension. Vasodilatation. Later bradycardia, negative inotropic action and hypotension.

      4. <u>Kidney</u>: Diuresis due to decreased vasopressin release.

      5. <u>Body temperature</u>: Poikilothermia-hypothermia.

      6. <u>Metabolic actions</u>: Initial slight hyperglycemia (catecholamine effect). Activation of kallikrein-increase in bradykinin. Increased plasma concentrations of high-density lipoproteins.

      7. <u>Endocrine actions</u>: Suppression of vasopressin secretion, increased ACTH, cortisol, and catecholamine secretion.

   B. Ethanol Absorption and Elimination:

      Approximately 30% of ethanol is absorbed from the stomach, and the remainder is rapidly absorbed from the small intestine. Ethanol is distributed according to tissue water content. Approximately 1-3% of ethanol is eliminated in the lungs (pulmonary blood/alveolar air ratio = 2100/1, the basis of breath tests), 2-6% is excreted by the kidney, and the remainder is oxidized in the liver at a constant rate. The total elimination rate is approximately 8-10 gms/hr, or 15-18 mg/100 ml blood/hr.

C. Disulfiram (Antabuse):

Disulfiram is an inhibitor of AlDH which can produce high blood levels of acetaldehyde after ethanol ingestion. Acetaldehyde syndrome includes skin flush (vasodilation), pulsating headache, dyspnea, nausea, sweating, chest pain, syncope, vertigo, blurred vision; possibly leading to hypotension and circulatory collapse in extreme cases. Clinically, disulfiram may be useful to reinforce the desire to stop drinking alcohol.

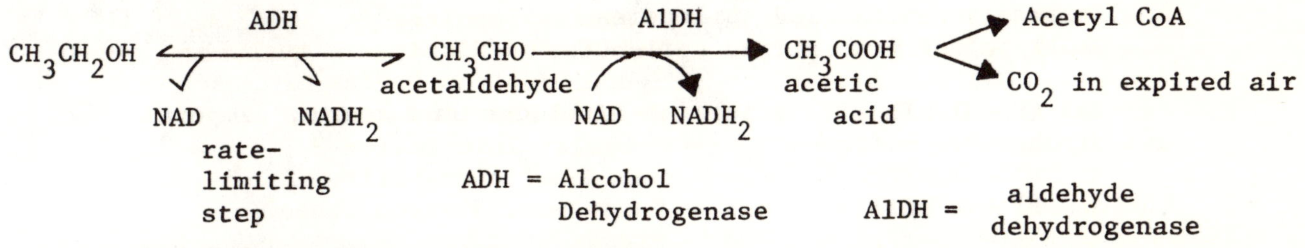

$$CH_3CH_2OH \xrightleftharpoons[NADH_2]{NAD}^{ADH} CH_3CHO \text{ (acetaldehyde)} \xrightarrow[NAD \quad NADH_2]{AlDH} CH_3COOH \text{ (acetic acid)} \longrightarrow \begin{cases} \text{Acetyl CoA} \\ CO_2 \text{ in expired air} \end{cases}$$

rate-limiting step

ADH = Alcohol Dehydrogenase

AlDH = aldehyde dehydrogenase

II. <u>Pathology of Chronic Ethanol Abuse</u>

1. <u>CNS Effects</u>: Wernicke's Syndrome, Korsakoff's psychosis, cerebral and cerebellar atrophy, alcoholic polyneuropathy (treated with thiamine)
2. <u>Gastrointestinal</u>: Peptic ulcers, esophagitis, gastritis and pancreatitis.
3. <u>Liver</u>: Steatosis, hepatitis, cirrhosis
4. <u>Muscle</u>: Cardiomyopathy, skeletal muscle myopathy
5. <u>Fetus</u>: Fetal alcohol syndrome

III. <u>Toxicology of Other Alcohols</u>

A. <u>Methanol</u>: Metabolized by ADH at about one-fifth the rate of ethanol to formaldehyde and then to formic acid. Toxicity due to metabolic acidosis and blindness caused by optic nerve damage. Treatment: Suppress methanol metabolism by administering ethanol; dialysis; bicarbonate to correct acidosis.

B. <u>Ethylene Glycol</u>: Metabolized to oxalic acid, causing systemic acidosis. Treatment same as for methanol.

ANTICONVULSANTS

Epilepsy (seizures, convulsive disorders): recurrent pattern of abnormal
discharges from brain neurons; may result in loss of consciousness or disturbances
of consciousness; changes in motor activity, behavior or sensory phenomena may
occur; site of neurons involved determines seizure pattern.

I.   Simplified – International Classification of the Epilepsies

   A.   Generalized seizures (bilaterally symmetrical and without local onset)

      1.   Primary generalized seizures (includes absences or petit mal,
           tonic-clonic or grand mal seizures, myoclonus and infantile spasms.
      2.   Secondary generalized epilepsies
      3.   Undetermined generalized epilepsies

   B.   Partial (focal, local) epilepsies (includes Jacksonian, temporal lobe,
        and psychomotor seizures

   C.   Unclassifiable epilepsies

Most seizures can be controlled by drugs; frequency and severity of seizures
reduced. Drug withdrawal initiated after two years of control except for
clonic-tonic-clonic seizures and clonic seizure of Janz where medication
must be taken for life.

II.   Spectrum

Seizure Type	Drug of First Choice (alone or in combination)	Alternate Drugs
Generalized tonic-clonic (grand mal) Partial cortical focal (including Jacksonian)	Phenytoin Phenobarbital Carbamazepine	Primidone Valproic acid
General absences (Petit mal)	Ethosuximide Valproic acid	Trimethadione
Partial complex (Temporal lobe, psychomotor)	Carbamazepine	Primidone Phenytoin
General myoclonus	Valproic acid	Clonazepam
General infantile spasms	Corticotropin (ACTH)	Clonazepam
Status epilepticus (i.v.) Continuous tonic-clonic	Diazepam (i.v.)	Phenytoin

III. Drugs

    A. <u>Phenytoin</u>: Variable bioavailability, Michaelis-Menten (saturation) <u>kinetics</u>, 90% protein bound; considerable inter-individual variation necessitating therapeutic monitoring, monitor more frequently during pregnancy. Adverse effects - nystagmus, ataxia, lethargy, and coma which are dose dependent. Gingival hyperplasia, hirsutism. Megaloblastic anemia which responds to folic acid; lupus-like syndrome and Stevens-Johnson Syndrome.

       Other uses - selected cardiac arrhythmias.

    B. <u>Phenobarbital</u>: Long acting barbiturate; well tolerated; induces microsomal enzymes; drowsiness, somnolence and ataxia are common; hyperexcitability in children; if a skin rash occurs after years of use - drug should be withdrawn because of danger of exfoliative dermatitis; abrupt withdrawal may precipitate seizures and lead to status epilepticus; withdraw slowly as other drugs are added to regimen.

    C. <u>Carbamazepine</u>: Chemically related to tricyclic antidepressants; autoinduction; active epoxide metabolite; drowsiness, ataxia, diploplia, gastric upset are common. Infrequently skin rashes, liver damage and bone marrow depression reported.

       Other uses - Trigeminal and glossopharyngeal neuralgias and selected forms of mania.

    D. <u>Ethosuximide</u>: A succinimide; side effects include sedation, drowsiness, headache and gastric upset; more serious and rare effects include blood dyscrasies, skin rashes, liver and kidney dysfunction.

    E. <u>Valproic Acid</u>: Widest spectrum; increases brain levels of GABA; gastric upset and sedation are common; hepatic toxicity and blood dyscrasias occur; must be monitored; increases incidence of spinal bifida in the fetus.

    F. <u>Primidone</u>: Metabolized to phenobarbital, sedation and ataxia occur even in low doses; other reactions include psychotic reactions, localized gingival pain, rashes and more rarely, megaloblastic anemia.

    G. <u>Trimethadione</u>: Used only if ethosuximide or valproic acid are ineffective in absences; causes sedation, ataxia, photosensitivity, hemeralopia, skin rashes and gastric upset; high incidence of serious side effects-kidney and liver damage, allergic dermatitis, agranulocytosis and aplastic anemia.

    H. <u>Clonazepam</u>: A benzodiazepine derivative; tolerance develops; ataxia, drowsiness and dysarthria commonly seen; behavioral or personality changes may be seen in children; blood dyscrasias are rare toxic effects.

    I. <u>Diazepam</u>: A benzodiazepine; used as <u>drug of choice i.v.</u> to terminate <u>status epilepticus</u> (seizures that last 30 minutes or longer or repeated seizures for 30 minutes or longer during which consciousness not regained - a medical emergency).

ANTIPARKINSONISM DRUGS

Parkinsonism is a degenerative disease of the CNS, characterized by the deficiency of dopamine in the striatal tracts. The resultant imbalance between the dopamine (inhibitory) and acetylcholine (excitatory) neurotransmitters leads to movement disorders. Therapy is therefore approached with dopaminergic or anticholinergic drugs, or with combinations of the two.

I. <u>Dopaminergic Drugs</u>

    A. <u>L-Dopa</u>: Penetrates into the CNS where it is decarboxylated to dopamine. The symptoms which respond most satisfactorily are bradykinesia and rigidity. Unpleasant side effects (nausea, vomiting, hypotension) early in therapy require slow increases in the dose of L-dopa. When L-dopa is combined with the peripheral decarboxylase inhibitor <u>carbidopa</u>, many of the peripheral side effects are diminished, and the L-dopa dosage can be reduced as much as 75%. Dyskinesias may be either a progression of the underlying disease or drug-induced. The philosophy of treatment has shifted towards the attainment of adequate function rather than the alleviation of all symptoms.

    B. <u>Amantadine</u>: An antiviral agent, the mechanism is attributed to a slow increased release of dopamine from storage sites. Amantadine is less effective than L-dopa, and its efficacy is diminished after 6 to 8 weeks of therapy. Therapy can be reinitiated once the stores are replenished.

    C. <u>Bromocriptine</u>: Is an agonist for the dopamine D-2 receptor.

        1. Not as effective as L-DOPA. The dose must be gradually increased to achieve optimal therapeutic effects. Primarily used to manage patients experiencing the "on-off" phenomena or as an adjunct if patients are not controlled with L-DOPA.

        2. Lowers elevated prolactin levels.

            a. Drug of choice for suppression of post-partum lactation, galactorrhea.

            b. Therapy of hyperprolactinemia for:

                i. amenorhea or oligomenorrhea

                ii. infertility

        3. Adjunct in therapy of acromegaly

    D. <u>Deprenyl</u>: Is a monoamine oxidase B inhibitor. Improvement may be brief.

II. <u>Anticholinergic drugs</u> (<u>trihexyphenidyl</u>, <u>benztropine</u> and others)

Primary use is in the treatment of mild symptoms or in combination therapy with L-dopa. Tremor responds most favorably to anticholinergics, and decreased salivary flow may diminish drooling. Anticholinergic side effects (e.g., urinary retention, constipation) often limit the usefulness of these drugs.

III. Known causes of Parkinson's disease

    A. Viruses

    B. Manganese toxicity

    C. Abuse of N-Methyl-4-phenyltetrahydropyridine (MPTP), an impurity found in illicit manufacturing of meperidine.

    D. Ischemia (stroke)

CNS MUSCLE RELAXANTS

DRUGS USED TO TREAT SKELETAL MUSCLE HYPERREACTIVITY

1. **Centrally Active Muscle Relaxants**

    a. <u>Baclofen</u> is the drug of choice for spinal spasticity, including multiple sclerosis. Baclofen is a derivative of gamma-aminobutyric acid (GABA) and may act as an agonist at bicuculline-insensitive GABA receptors (GABA$_B$), localized primarily in laminae II and III of the spinal cord dorsal horn. The dosage is slowly increased to reach maximum therapeutic effectiveness. Excreted is largely unchanged-caution with renal impairment. Side effects include drowsiness, GI symptoms and muscle weakness. Abrupt termination of baclofen therapy may cause anxiety and hallucinations, so the drug is gradually discontinued.

    b. <u>Diazepam</u> is the most commonly used benzodiazepine for the therapy of spinal spasticity, although all sedative-hypnotics which decrease internuncial transmission may be equally effective. Tolerance develops, if used in chronic conditions. Drug holidays should be interspersed between courses of therapy.

    c. <u>Cyclobenzaprine</u> is structurally related to the tricyclic antidepressant, amitriptyline, but has no mood elevation effects; tolerance develops; used in acute trauma; side effects are drowiness, dry mouth and dizziness.

    d. Other centrally-acting muscle relaxants (carisprodol, methocarbamol, etc.) are used primarily for the treatment of acute muscle spasms. Their clinical effectiveness has been difficult to establish, and their activity may be largely due to their sedative effects.

2. **Locally Active Muscle Relaxants**

    <u>Dantrolene</u> interferes with calcium efflux in muscle cells, and has no effect on neural pathways. Dantrolene provides significant and sustained relief of symptoms in many paraplegic and hemiplegic patients, but is less effective than baclofen in multiple sclerosis. Common side effects are drowsiness, nausea and muscle weakness.

    Fatal hepatotoxicity has occurred with long term dantrolene therapy and with high doses. Patients receiving long-term dantrolene therapy should be monitored for hepatic damage (e.g., SGOT, SGPT).

    Dantrolene is the drug of choice in the treatment of malignant hyperthermia, and is given i.v. when the symptoms are first recognized.

CNS STIMULANTS

A. Drugs that can produce convulsions

    1. <u>Strychnine</u>: acts on spinal cord by blocking glycine-induced postsynaptic inhibition; treat convulsions with barbiturates.
    2. <u>Picrotoxin</u>: acts on brain stem by blocking GABA mediated presynaptic inhibition.
    3. <u>Pentylenetetrazol</u>: acts on brainstem; mechanism unknown; used in past for convulsive therapy.
    4. <u>Miscellaneous Analeptics</u>: <u>doxapram</u> and <u>ethamivan</u>; used in past to treat barbiturate overdose; now treatment of choice for barbiturate overdose is to support respiration and the cardiovascular system.

B. Psychomotor stimulants

Amphetamines (A)
Methylphenidate (M)
Cocaine (C)

    1. <u>Mechanism</u>: indirect-acting adrenergic agents (A,M,C); some MAO inhibition (A); intraneuronal release of catecholamines (A,M); blockade of catecholamine reuptake (A,M,C); these actions result in an increase in the concentration of catecholamines at the adrenoceptors.

    2. <u>CNS stimulant effects</u>: mood elevation, wakefulness, decreased sense of fatigue, euphoria, hallucinations, appetite suppression, alteration in time perception, generalized increase in motor activity (including agitation).

    3. <u>Cardiovascular</u>: increased systolic and diastolic pressure that may be accompanied by reflex bradycardia, cardiac arrhythmias due to catecholamine release.

    4. <u>Smooth muscle</u>: slight bronchial relaxant effect, variable effects on GI motility.

    5. <u>Toxicity</u>: restlessness, tremors, irritability, headache, sleep disturbances, fatigue, depression, hallucinations, paranoid behavior, aggressive behavior, arterial aneurysms, necrotizing angiitis.

    6. <u>Therapeutic uses</u>: narcolepsy, hyperkinetic and perceptually handicapped children; controversial in the treatment of obesity.

    7. <u>Metabolism</u>:

        a. Majority of amphetamine is not metabolized.
            i. increased excretion in an acidic urine.
           ii. what is metabolized is handled by oxidative deamination.
        b. Cocaine is metabolized in both liver and in plasma. Hepatic damage may occur, due to toxic metabolites.

C. Xanthines

Caffeine, theophylline, theobromine, pentoxifylline

1. <u>Mechanism</u>: adenosine receptor antagonists, increases intracellular calcium; high doses may increase cyclic AMP by inhibiting phosphodiesterase, .

2. <u>CNS</u>: increased alertness and motor activity, decreased fatigue and drowiness, respiratory stimulation, may interfer with sleep.

3. <u>Other systems</u>: Increases gastric secretions which may be important in etiology of reflux esophagitis; constriction of cerebral vasculature, relaxation of smooth muscle except cerebrovascular; dilation of coronary, pulmonary and peripheral vasculature; large dose may produce direct myocardial stimulation.

4. <u>Toxicity</u>: Insomnia, restlessness, muscle tremors, convulsion (especially in asthmatics).

5. <u>Therapeutic uses</u>: Bronchial asthma (theophylline) and vasodilating headaches (caffeine); apnea in the newborn infant (caffeine, theophylline); intermittent claudication due to chronic occlusive arterial disease (pentoxifylline).

6. <u>Pentoxifylline</u>:

   a. Highly bound to erthyrocyte, active metabolites.
   b. Hemorheological effect (improve capillary blood flow).

      i. increasing erthyrocytic flexibility via inhibition of 3',5' adenosine monophosphate diesterase, which increases cyclic AMP in RBC.
      ii. decrease in viscosity of blood by:

         1. reduced platelet aggregation by increase synthesis release of prostacyclin (PGI_2)
         2. reduction in fibrinogin in blood

ANTIDEPRESSANTS

A. Psychomotor stimulants: NOT CLINICALLY APPROPRIATE AS ANTIDEPRESSANTS.

B. Tricyclic antidepressants: Drugs of choice in treatment of depression.
Examples:

1. Imipramine
2. Desipramine
3. Amitriptyline
4. Doxepine
    Mechanism of therapeutic effect in CNS unknown; cocaine-like action in
    preventing reuptake of catecholamines; also have atropine-like actions
    thus should be used cautiously in patients with glaucoma; no physical or
    psychic dependence; do not co-administer with MAO inhibitors, wait at
    least 1 week to avoid the possibility of a hypertensive crisis.

    Imipramine and amitryptyline are the oldest tricyclic antidepressants and
    the newer tricyclics have not been clearly shown to be superior. Doxepine
    is advertised as differing from the other tricyclics in that it does not
    block the antihypertensive actions of guanethidine (a cocaine-like
    effect). There are now a number of clinically useful antidepressants
    which do not have cocaine like effects (that is: blockade of
    norepinephrine re-uptake by nerve terminals).

    Doxepine and amitryptyline are considered to be the most sedative and
    protriptyline the least sedative. For this reason it has been suggested
    that doxepine be used in cases of mixed anxiety-depression.

    Amitriptyline is the most potent anticholinergic and desipramine is the
    least.

    REMEMBER: Side effects from tricyclics can begin with the first dosing.
    Therapeutic response can be delayed for as long as 3 weeks.

Side Effects:

1. Anticholinergic side effects include: dry mouth, blurred vision,
    constipation, tachycardia and urinary retention.
2. Other types of side effects include: obstructive jaundice, seizures (high
    doses), hallucinations, agranulocytosis, and drug interactions.
3. Symptoms of accidental overdosage, often seen in the children of depressed
    patients taking their parents medication are: hyperpyrexia, hypertension,
    seizures, and coma.
4. Treatment of overdoses includes: gastric lavage, symptomatic treatment
    and physostigmine for CNS anticholinergic effects.

C. Second-generation antidepressants: Trazadone is the only one extensively
used, relatively free of anticholinergic adverse effects, marked sedative
actions, priapism-has limited use in males. Maprotiline: on high or rapidly
escalating doses has high incidence of seizures.

D. MAO inhibitors: Inhibition of monoamine oxidase and a variety of other
enzymes, thus are very toxic and long acting. Examples: 1) isocarboxazid, 2)

phenelzine, 3) <u>tranylcypromine</u>, 4) <u>pargyline</u>. Increase Epi, NE, 5-HT, and
dopamine in brain; potentiate actions of other drugs such as alcohol and
narcotics (probably via inhibition of hepatic enzymes); may take several weeks
for MAO levels to return to normal upon cessation of treatment; do not use at
same time with tricyclic antidepressants; used only in patients refractory to
tricyclic antidepressant drugs. Patients treated with MAO inhibitors may
develop severe <u>hypertension</u> after eating foods that contain <u>tyramine</u>. May
produce hepatotoxic effects in some patients.

<u>DRUGS USED IN THE TREATMENT OF MANIC-DEPRESSIVE DISORDERS</u>

<u>Lithium salts</u>: Mimics sodium in body fluids; excreted by kidneys; caution should
be used in decreasing daily sodium intake or the use of diuretics in the
management of hypertension in patients stablized on a daily lithium dose (may
result in toxic blood levels of lithium); mechanism of action not known; tends to
decrease the amplitude of the manic-depressive mood swings. Administered orally
and may produce GI irritation. Has a long plasma $t\frac{1}{2}$ (renal excretion).
Significant alteration in dietary sodium ($\downarrow$ or $\uparrow$) can interfere with therapy.
Significant toxicity (above 1.5 mEq/L) includes lethargy, muscle fasciculations,
cardiac arrhythmias and seizures. <u>NO ANTIDOTE EXISTS</u>

ANTI-PSYCHOTICS

<u>Anti-psychotic drugs</u>: Are effective in the treatment of psychoses; improve symptoms of psychotic mental disease; they are not a "cure" in themselves; treatment must be individualized and some may require indefinite and uninterrupted treatment; there may be large individual differences in daily dosage required for therapeutic effect.

A. <u>Phenothiazine derivatives</u>: Used in the treatment of psychotic patients. In addition, these drugs can be used in the management of organic psychiatric disorders, movement disorders and intractable hiccough and alcohol withdrawal hallucinosis. They have been used in the treatment of nausea and vomiting of pregnancy and other forms of chemically induced nausea and vomiting (effective competitive blockade of chemoreceptor trigger zone (CTZ) in medulla; this area sends neurons to the "vomiting center"; phenothiazines effective only in emesis induced by this mechanism, i.e., by compounds such as morphine, apomorphine, digitalis glycosides and aspirin in high doses). Major side effects include hypotension (tolerance develops) and extrapyramidal effects that include AKINESIA, AKATHASIA, DYSTONIA and DYSKINESIA (tolerance does not develop here). The CNS potency parallels the anti-emetic action and also the extrapyramidal effects.

1. <u>Piperazine</u> side chain most potent. Examples: <u>Trifluoperazine</u> and perphenazine. 2. <u>Piperidine</u> compounds least potent, i.e., <u>Thioridazine</u>. 3. Aliphatic types are intermediate, i.e., <u>Chlorpromazine</u>.

<u>Chlorpromazine</u> (prototype): Sedative action when first administered (Neuroleptic syndrome, tolerance develops over time); impairs conditioned responses (basis for screening these compounds); does not depress respiration and is not analgesic at clinical doses; blocks CTZ (i.e., blocks emesis to apomorphine but not that due to $CuSO_4$ which acts as an irritant of the gastic mucosa and does not directly stimulate the CTZ); strong adrenergic and weak cholinergic blocking properties; hypotension (some tolerance here over time—mainly a CNS effect); oral or parenteral; long sojourn in body; not addicting, no physical dependence, no euphoria; toxic reactions include: 1. hypersensitivity: most dangerous, 2. jaundice: usually obstructive type, 3. weight gain, 4. photosensitivity, 5. dryness of mouth and blurred vision, 6. extrapyramidal side effects and orthostatic hypotension; these agents also have some anti-histamine actions, 7. agranulocytosis and leukopenia can occur, 8. increased prolactin levels (gynecomastia) and decreased ACTH, testosterone, estrogen and other steroids.

B. <u>Thioxanthenes</u>: Carbon rather than nitrogen in ring structure; otherwise much like phenothiazines

1. Aliphatic: <u>Chlorprothixene</u>; structure like chlorpromazine.
2. Piperazine: <u>Thiothixene</u>.

C. <u>Butyrophenones</u>: i.e., <u>Haloperidol</u>; similar in action to piperazine substituted phenothiazines; same therapeutic indications and side effects. Potent dopamine receptor blockers with a <u>high incidence</u> of extrapyramidal reactions and tardive dyskinesias.

D. <u>Primozide</u>: Similar in action to haloperidol.

<u>OPIOID ANALGESICS</u>

1. <u>Functional classification of narcotic opioids</u>:

    a. Narcotic analgesics: morphine, oxycodone, methadone, meperidine,
        fentanyl, codeine and propoxyphene.
    b. Narcotic antagonists: naloxone and naltrexone.
    c. Mixed agonist-antagonists: butorphanol, nalbuphine and pentazocine.
    d. Antitussives: codeine and dextromethorphan.

2. <u>Proposed mechanisms</u>:

    Opiate analgesics interact with endogenous receptors.

    The natural agonist for these receptors has been proposed to be the
    opiate-like peptides.

    There are three generally recognized groups of opioid peptides:

    a. Endorphins
    b. Enkephalins
    c. Dynorphans

    Data to date indicates that these peptides represent distinct groups of gene
    products, i.e., pre-prodynorphan is a completely different compound from
    pre-proenkephalin. Similarly, these precursor molecules have different
    messenger RNA's.

    There are probably 20 or more peptides present in nature (even within a single
    organism) that can interact with one or more of the opiate receptors.

    Consistent with multiple opiate peptides, there are multiple opiate receptors.

<u>Receptor</u>	<u>Agonist</u>	<u>Function</u>
<u>Mu</u>	Morphine	Analgesia etc.
<u>Kappa</u>	Benzomorphans	Analgesia in spinal cord and above
<u>Sigma</u>	Benzomorphans	Adverse psychological effects
<u>Delta</u>	Methionine enkephalin	Analgesia produced by peptides

3. <u>Basic properties of narcotic analgesics: Morphine is the prototype.</u>

    a. <u>Analgesia</u>: selective effect; best against pain of visceral origin;
        multiple sites of action; increases in threshold to pain, alters central
        reception or perception of pain information, depresses the patient's
        reaction to pain. (Remember that in the treatment of pain there is a
        significant placebo effect).
    b. <u>Euphoria</u> is independent of analgesia; of patients given morphine 75%
        experience euphoria and 25% experience dysphoria.

c. <u>Sedative</u> (narcosis means to promote sleep). Sedation is a secondary action of analgesics.

d. <u>Anti-tussive</u>: depresses the cough reflex center in the medulla; not a specific narcotic effect.

e. <u>Respiratory depression</u>: limits the therapeutic use (especially in patients with abnormal curvature of the spine and in obese patients).

f. <u>Emetic action</u>: initial dose stimulates the chemoreceptor emetic trigger zone (CTZ). In ambulatory patients, 40% get nauseous, 20% vomit. Subsequent doses block vomiting by depression of the vomiting center.

g. <u>Miosis</u> (pinpoint pupils): stimulation of Edinger-Westphal nucleus (oculomotor nucleus) in human; some animals (cat, monkey) have mydriasis.

h. <u>Convulsant action</u>: can stimulate cortex or spinal cord to get strychnine-like convulsions; rare in humans.

i. <u>Histamine release</u>: frequently seen after I.V. injection. Because of the histamine release effect, patients may complain of "itching", particularly after morphine.

j. <u>Constipating effect</u>: 1) increases tone and decreases propulsive activity throughout intestinal tract and 2) increases tone of anal sphincter and depresses (abolishes) defecation reflex; increases tone of various sphincters (biliary colic).

k. <u>Tolerance</u>: develops to most of morphine effects; exceptions are constipation and central stimulatory effects (including miosis). <u>Cross-tolerance</u> develops to other narcotic analgesics.

l. <u>Neuroendocrine changes</u>: inhibition of release of ACTH and consequent reduction in 17-hydroxysteroids; release of adrenal epinephrine and consequent hyperglycemia.

5. <u>Other useful narcotic analgesia</u>:
<u>Codeine</u>: a specific narcotic analgesic with therapeutically significant antitussive effects; sedation is unusual, excitement may occur and large doses may cause convulsions. Well absorbed orally.
<u>Meperidine</u>: pupillary size and pupillary reflex either are not affected or mydriasis may occur. Its metabolite, normeperidine, may produce convulsions.
<u>Fentanyl</u>: about 50-80 times more potent than morphine; respiratory depression is of shorter duration than with meperidine.
<u>Propoxyphene</u>: 65 mg is equivalent to 600 mg of aspirin.

6. <u>Withdrawal</u>: with morphine, heroin, codeine, peak abstinence at 36-72 hours; meperidine, 7-12 hours; methadone, about 7 days. <u>Early symptoms</u> (10-12 hours) include: rhinorrhea, perspiration, lacrimation, and yawning. <u>Intermediate symptoms</u> (18-24 hours); mydriasis, piloerection, anorexia, muscular tremors. <u>Peak symptoms</u> (36-72 hours); restlessness, hot flashes alternating with chills, increase in blood pressure and heart rate, increase in rate and depth of respiration, fever 1° or more, nausea, retching, vomiting and diarrhea. Withdrawal from a narcotic is generally not life threatening although almost unbearable.

7. <u>Narcotic antagonists</u>: can immediately reverse all of the depressant effects of the opiates and some of the stimulatory effects, such as vomiting, miosis, hypothermia, bradycardia, and gastrointestinal spasm, but not convulsions and probably not the antitussive effect. Signs of withdrawal appear in 5-15 minutes, reach a peak in 30-45 minutes, and last only a few hours but are very, very intensive. <u>Naloxone</u> is the clinically available antagonist. The $t_{\frac{1}{2}}$ for naloxone is sufficiently shorter than morphine so that repetitive doses

may be necessary to adequately block the depressant effects of morphine and other narcotics. Naltrexone has a longer $t_\frac{1}{2}$.

8. <u>Partial agonist:</u>
<u>Pentazocine</u>: is a partial agonist or mixed agonist - antagonist analgesic which can be used in treating mild to moderate pain. Because it does have antagonist activity it should never be used as an analgesic in physically dependent patients (including methadone maintenance). It is reported to have a much lower abuse liability than the other narcotics used to treat moderate pain.

9. <u>Antitussives</u>: Dextromethorphan can be considered a prototype. It suppresses coughing through central mechanisms not well understood. It elevates the threshold for coughing. In therapeutic doses, it produces little, if any, gastrointestinal disturbance or sedation. High doses may produce respiratory depression. It does not show cross-tolerance with morphine and its actions are not modified by narcotic antagonists. Its therapeutic use should be considered as a very low risk with regard to liability to abuse.

HALLUCINOGENIC DRUGS

1. A wide variety of CNS active compounds may produce hallucinatory effects either as a primary effect or as a secondary (side) effect. Emotional lability is a common presenting symptom.

2. Chemical classes represented include:

    a. Ergot alkaloids

        Prototype: LSD-25

    b. Tryptamine derivatives

        Psilocybin
        Psilocin
        Dimethyltryptamine (DMT, "Business-man's trip")

    c. Phenylalkylamine derivatives

        MDA
        MDMA (Ecstasy)
        MDEA
        Mescaline
        DOM (STP)

    d. Anticholinergics

        Scopolamine
        Atropine
        Tricyclic antidepressants (especially in elderly)

    e. Miscellaneous compounds

        Phencyclidine (angel dust; often sold as "THC crystal")
        Δ^9 THC

3. On a relative potency basis:

    LSD > psilocybin > mescaline

    They all appear to have a common mechanism of action.

4. No one neurotransmitter system appears to be involved. The development of physical dependence with these drugs is difficult to demonstrate (if at all).

5. In the treatment of phencyclidine intoxication, acidification of the urine will _greatly_ enhance the rate of clearance. This can be accomplished by giving ammonium chloride or in a pinch, even ascorbic acid in large doses should have some effect.

6. Antipsychotic drugs (e.g. chlorpromazine) are useful in managing the drug intoxication.

DRUG ABUSE

Essentially all drugs that can produce euphoria have been abused. These include narcotic drugs; CNS stimulants (amphetamines and cocaine), CNS depressants - (alcohol, barbiturates, non-barbiturate sedative-hypnotics, antianxiety drugs and inhalants, such as amyl nitrite, or solvents such as toluene, benzene, acetone, carbon tetrachloride), hallucinogenic or psychotominetic drugs (lysergic acid derivatives, tryptamine derivatives, mescaline, cannabis, and miscellaneous compounds such as Freon[R] and myristicin [Nutmeg]).

Drugs of abuse can be divided into groups, according to whether they produce both physical dependence and psychological dependence or whether they produce only psychological dependence.

PHYSICAL AND PSYCHOLOGICAL DEPENDENCE		PSYCHOLOGICAL DEPENDENCE	
Narcotics	morphine heroin methadone meperidine codeine dextropropoxyphene	Stimulants	amphetamine cocaine caffeine
		Nicotine	
Sedative/Hypnotics	ethanol pentobarbital secobarbital diazepam chlordiazepoxide	Hallucinogens	mescaline LSD Δ^9-THC MDMA Phencyclidine
		Miscellaneous	nitrous oxide gasoline amyl nitrite Freon*

*May cause "freezing of the airway" and halogenated hydrocarbons may sensitize the myocardium to catecholamine-induced arrhythmia.

REVIEW QUESTIONS

<u>ONE BEST ANSWER</u>

1. _______ Side effects which can result from the administration of a narcotic analgesic drug, such as morphine, include all of the following EXCEPT:

    1. Urinary retention
    2. Nausea and vomiting
    3. Diarrhea
    4. Dysphoria
    5. Constriction of bronchiolar smooth muscle

2. _______ Among the hallucinogens, psilocybin, mescaline and LSD, one might expect them to differ in which one of the following characteristics?

    1. Development of tolerance
    2. Development of cross tolerance
    3. Potency
    4. Nature of the hallucinations
    5. Psychological effects

3. _______ Antianxiety drugs and antipsychotics share which side effect?

    1. Physical dependence
    2. Sedation
    3. Extrapyramidal symptoms
    4. Antiemetic action
    5. Muscle-relaxant activity

4. _______ The predominant process responsible for terminating the central depressant action of a single dose of pentobarbital is which one of the following?

    1. Metabolic degradation
    2. Renal excretion
    3. Physical redistribution
    4. None of the above

5. _______ The systemic manifestations of a serious toxic reaction to a local anesthetic agent includes some combination of the following: hypotension, respiratory depression and/or convulsions. The most probable cause is:

    1. Psychogenic
    2. Deterioration of the anesthetic agent
    3. Patient hypersensitivity to the vasoconstrictor
    4. Excessive blood level of the anesthetic agent
    5. Patient hypersensitivity to the anesthetic agent

<u>ONE BEST ANSWER</u>

6. _______ The physical constant of general anesthetic agents that determines the rate of induction and rate of recovery is:

    1. Lipid solubility
    2. Binding to tissue protein
    3. Diffusion capacity relative to oxygen
    4. Blood-gas solubility coefficient

7. _______ Tonic-clonic seizures with hypocapnia are a potential adverse effect associated with which one of the following inhalation anesthetic agents?

    1. Nitrous oxide
    2. Halothane
    3. Enflurane
    4. Isoflurane

8. _______ Degeneration of the nasal septum is most often associated with abuse of:

    1. LSD
    2. Ethyl alcohol
    3. Amphetamine
    4. Cocaine

9. _______ Which one of the following compounds produces Parkinsonism?

    1. Amphetamine
    2. Ecstasy (MDMA)
    3. DMT (Dimethyltryptamine)
    4. MPTP (Methylphenyltetrahydropyridine)

10. _______ Catecholamine-induced cardiac arrhythmias following exposure to halogenated hydrocarbon are associated with the abuse of which one of the following compounds?

    1. Naptha
    2. Xylene
    3. Benzene
    4. Freon

11. _______ Lithium overdose is best treated by:

    1. Chelation of the lithium with EDTA
    2. Administration of protamine to complex with the lithium
    3. Termination of the dosing
    4. Removal of the lithium by frequent gastic lavage

<u>ONE BEST ANSWER</u>

12. _______   The analgesic efficiacy is greatest for:

1. Aspirin
2. Acetaminophen
3. Aspirin + Acetaminophen
4. Codeine
5. Codeine + Aspirin

13. _______   Relief of tooth pain by oxycodone is due to:

1. Inhibition of nerve transmission in the tooth pulp
2. Reduction in edema and local inflammatory reactions
3. Inhibition of prostaglandin synthesis
4. Activation of narcotic receptors in spinal cord and brain

14. _______   Central excitement associated with inebriation from ethanol is the result of?

1. Irritation of sensory endings in the throat and stomach
2. Direct stimulation of cortical centers
3. Amnesia
4. Depression of higher centers of the central nervous system
5. Stimulation of internuncial neurons in the spinal cord

15. _______   An antitussive effect is produced by all of the following EXCEPT:

1. Codeine
2. Dihydrocodeine
3. Dextromethorphan
4. Diphenhydramine
5. Morphine

16. _______   Antipsychotic effects of chlorpromazine are thought to be caused by the blockade of which receptor system?

1. Limbic serotonin
2. Striatal dopamine
3. Striatal enkephalin
4. Limbic dopamine

17. _______   Administered orally, theophylline is the most potent of the methylxanthines in producing all of the following effects EXCEPT:

1. Direct stimulation of the myocardium
2. Dilation of the coronary arteries
3. Relaxation of bronchial smooth muscle
4. Stimulation of the central nervous system
5. Promoting diuresis

<u>ONE BEST ANSWER</u>

18. _______ Treatment of acute poisoning by sedative-hypnotics include all of the following EXCEPT:

1. Maintain the airway, assist ventilation if required
2. Prevent acidosis
3. Give a general CNS stimulant
4. Give a specific antagonist if available
5. Support the circulation and maintain body temperature

19. _______ The drug of choice for the treatment of malignant hyperthermia is:

1. Diazepam
2. Caffeine
3. Halothane
4. Baclofen
5. Dantrolene

20. _______ Acute intermittent porphyria is an absolute contraindication for the use of which group of drugs:

1. Stimulants
2. Psychotherapeutic drugs
3. Anti-parkinson's drugs
4. Barbiturates
5. Dantrolene

21. _______ An anticholinergic drug is the drug of choice for treating which one of the primary symptoms of Parkinson's disease?

1. Rigidity
2. Akinesthesia and bradykinesthesia
3. Shuffling gait
4. Tremor

22. _______ Bromocriptine is:

1. A peripheral decarboxylase inhibitor
2. A dopamine receptor agonist
3. A dopamine releaser
4. Monoamine oxidase B inhibitor

23. _______ The prime difference between alprazolam and triazolam is:

1. Efficacy
2. Potency
3. Slope of the dose-response curves
4. Individual variability
5. Marketing

<u>ONE BEST ANSWER</u>

24. _______ The CNS syndromes associated with alcoholism are considered primarily
to be caused by which one of the following:

1. Direct toxicity of ethanol
2. Direct toxicity of acetaldehyde
3. Inflammatory effects of alcohol
4. Malnutrition

25. _______ Biliary colic is often severe with meperidine compared to morphine
because:

1. Meperidine is not absorbed orally
2. Morphine is metabolized to codeine which produces colic
3. Meperidine has antiserotonergic effects
4. Meperidine has antimuscarinic effects

26. _______ The current drug of choice in treating hyperkinetic and perceptually
handicapped children is:

1. Theophylline
2. Phenobarbital
3. Methylphenidate
4. Diazepam

27. _______ Which one of the following is most likely to produce an increase in
pulmonary arterial pressure?

1. Codeine
2. Butorphanol
3. Methadone
4. Morphine

28. _______ Although inhalation general anesthetics have low therapeutic indices,
their clinical safety is enhanced because of:

1. Rapid liver metabolism
2. Specific antagonists
3. Rapid renal excretion
4. Rapid tissue redistribution
5. Low bioavailability

29. _______ In anesthesiology what is MAC (minimum alveolar concentration)?

1. Lethal dose
2. Median lethal dose
3. Anesthetic dose
4. Median effective dose

<u>ONE BEST ANSWER</u>

30. _______ During the establishment of an adequate daily phenytoin dose, small
increases in dose are often required in the therapeutic range. The
primary pharmacological reason is:

1. Poor oral absorption of phenytoin
2. A change in extent of protein binding
3. Saturation of the enzyme involved in phenytoin metabolism
4. An alteration in the affinity of the phenytoin receptor

31. _______ The therapeutic use of diazepam in epilepsy is associated with which
disorder:

1. Generalized tonic-clonic seizures
2. Absences
3. Partial seizures with complex symptomatology
4. Febrile seizures
5. Status epilepticus

32. _______ Forced diuresis and alkalinization of the urine would speed the
excretion of:

1. Amphetamine
2. Phenytoin
3. Aspirin
4. Morphine

33. _______ The most potent hallucinogen is:

1. LSD-25
2. Mescaline
3. Amphetamine
4. <u>delta</u>^{9}-Tetrahydrocannabinol
5. Bufotenin

34. _______ All of the following statements about amphetamine are true EXCEPT:

1. May produce a lethal hypertensive crisis
2. Improves learning ability
3. At high doses may produce a "paranoid-like" psychosis
4. Reduces fatigue
5. Improves performance of well-learned behaviors

35. _______ Naloxone is useful in the emergency treatment of respiratory
depression produced by:

1. Alcohol
2. Chlorpromazine
3. Codeine
4. Diazepam
5. Phencyclidine

MULTIPLE TRUE-FALSE

Directions: For each of the statements below, ONE or MORE of the completions given is correct.

       1 - If only 1, 2 and 3 are correct
       2 - If only 1 and 3 are correct
       3 - If only 2 and 4 are correct
       4 - If only 4 is correct
       5 - If all are correct

36. _______ The most efficacious antidepressant(s) are:

1. Imipramine
2. Desipramine
3. Amitriptylline
4. Doxepin

37. _______ Side effects from tricyclic antidepressants include:

1. Dry mouth
2. Urinary retention
3. Blurred vision
4. Parkinsonian-like effects

38. _______ The effects of imipramine are terminated by:

1. Urinary excretion of unchanged drug
2. Hepatic microsomal metabolism to desipramine
3. Urinary excretion of metabolites
4. Exhalation from lungs

39. _______ Extrapyramidal reactions following doses of antipsychotics are:

1. Due to dopamine receptor blockade in the extrapyramidal system
2. Due to acetylcholine receptor blockade in the extrapyramidal system
3. Reversed by CNS cholinergic antagonists
4. Blocked by CNS dopamine antagonists

40. _______ Pharmacological effects of the barbiturates and benzodiazepines include:

1. Sedation
2. Muscle relaxation
3. Anticonvulsant action
4. Physical dependence

41. _______ The benzodiazepine receptor works in concert with:

1. Dopamine receptor
2. Gamma aminobutyric acid (GABA) receptor
3. Sodium ionophore
4. Chloride ionophore

<u>MULTIPLE TRUE - FALSE</u>
Directions Summarized:

1	2	3	4	5
1,2,3 only	1,3 only	2,4 only	4 only	all are correct

42. _______ In case of acute overdose with pentazocine the most important therapeutic measure is to:

    1. Give doxapram
    2. Give naloxone
    3. Give caffeine
    4. Maintain respiration

43. _______ Withdrawal from a sedative-hypnotic can be characterized by:

    1. Tonic-clonic (grand mal) seizures
    2. Toxic psychosis
    3. Cardiovascular collapse
    4. Precipitation by pentazocine

44. _______ Compared with ether, nitrous oxide has:

    1. Poor analgesic effect
    2. Pronounced muscle relaxation
    3. Prominent respiratory depression effect
    4. A lower Ostwald partition coefficient and potency

45. _______ The following apply to the phenomenon of tolerance to narcotic analgesics:

    1. Tolerance develops faster with large doses given at short intervals, than with small doses given at longer intervals
    2. Tolerance develops at the same rate for all the actions of narcotic analgesics
    3. An individual tolerant to morphine will also be tolerant to meperidine and methadone
    4. Once acquired, tolerance is lost only after several weeks of drug abstinence

46. _______ Withdrawal signs occur after cessation of chronic use of:

    1. Meperidine
    2. Secobarbital
    3. Alcohol
    4. Marihuana

47. _______ Disulfiram inhibits:

    1. Dopamine-beta hydroxylase
    2. Xanthine oxidase
    3. Acetaldehyde dehydrogenase
    4. Alcohol dehydrogenase

<u>MULTIPLE TRUE – FALSE</u>
<u>Directions Summarized:</u>

1	2	3	4	5
1,2,3 only	1,3 only	2,4 only	4 only	all are correct

48. _______ Which of the following agents could decrease the patient's reaction to pain?

1. Analgesics
2. Sedatives
3. Tranquilizers
4. Placebos

49. _______ Chlorpromazine can cause:

1. Blood dyscrasias
2. "Obstructive" jaundice
3. Postural hypotension
4. Photosensitization

50. _______ Which of the following drugs are useful for muscle relaxation due to an acute injury?

1. Phenobarbital
2. Cyclobenzaprine
3. Diazepam
4. Buspirone

51. _______ Which of the following measures may be necessary in the treatment of toxic reactions due to local anesthetic overdosage:

1. Administration of diazepam
2. Administration of O_2
3. Artificial respiration
4. Administration of i.v. fluids and vasoconstrictor agents

52. _______ Epinephrine is included in many local anesthetic preparations because it:

1. Prolongs the period of anesthesia
2. Increases the activity of plasma esterases
3. Reduces the systemic toxicity of local anesthetics
4. Prevents allergic reactions

53. _______ Diazepam is the drug of choice for which of the following parasomnias:

1. Sleep walking
2. Sleep walking with complex and, at times, violent behavior
3. Night terrors
4. Primary enuresis

<u>MULTIPLE TRUE - FALSE</u>
Directions Summarized:

1	2	3	4	5
1,2,3	1,3	2,4	4	all are
only	only	only	only	correct

54. _______ Parkinson's disease is characterized by:

1. Tremor
2. Increased salivation and dysphagia
3. Paralysis of facial muscles
4. Rigidity

55. _______ In manganese toxicity there is a DECREASE in striatal dopamine levels; rational therapy could include treatment with which of the following drugs:

1. Anticholinergic drug
2. Chlorpromazine
3. L-DOPA
4. Haloperidol

56. _______ Naloxone has:

1. High affinity for the Mu narcotic receptor
2. Low affinity for the Mu narcotic receptor
3. Low intrinsic activity
4. High intrinsic activity

57. _______ "Recreational" misuse of nitrous oxide might lead to a neuropathy characterized by:

1. Distal numbness
2. Weakness
3. Incoordination
4. Amnesia

58. _______ The shorter-acting benzodiazepines include:

1. Flurazepam
2. Triazolam
3. Chlordiazepoxide
4. Oxazepam

59. _______ Hydroxyzine:

1. Is often combined with chloral hydrate
2. Is a benzodiazepine
3. Has antiemetic properties
4. Has anticonvulsant properties

MULTIPLE TRUE - FALSE
Directions Summarized:

1	2	3	4	5
1,2,3 only	1,3 only	2,4 only	4 only	all are correct

60. _______ Carbamazepine is used to treat:

1. Pain from cancer
2. Trigeminal neuralgias
3. Multiple sclerosis
4. Partial seizures with complex symptomatology

61. _______ The action of baclofen is associated with which receptor(s):

1. Adenosine
2. $GABA_A$
3. Mu
4. $GABA_B$

62. _______ An appropriate induction anesthetic for high risk patients or neurosurgical patients with increased intracranial pressure would be:

1. Etomidate
2. Diazepam
3. Midazolam
4. Thiopental

63. _______ In man, morphine is metabolized by:

1. N-acetylation
2. Glucuronidation
3. Sulfoxidation
4. N-dealkylation

64. _______ Overdoses of imipramine are treated by which of the following methods:

1. Gastric lavage
2. Neostigmine
3. Physostigmine
4. Intravenous lithium

65. _______ Increased prolactin concentrations are seen with which of the following:

1. Haloperidol
2. Trifluoperazine
3. Thioridazine
4. Doxepin

<u>MULTIPLE TRUE - FALSE</u>
<u>Directions Summarized:</u>

1	2	3	4	5
1,2,3	1,3	2,4	4	all are
only	only	only	only	correct

66. _______ Enhanced performance of learned tasks is associated with:

    1. Amphetamine
    2. Cocaine
    3. Caffeine
    4. Ethanol

67. _______ Tardive dyskinesias:

    1. Never occur if the dose of haloperidol is above 5 mg/day
    2. Are due to hypersensitivity of the cholinergic system
    3. Are always permanent neurologic changes
    4. Are more likely to occur in patients who have acute
        extrapyramidal reactions with the antipsychotic

68. _______ Antipsychotic-induced extrapyramidal reactions include:

    1. Catatonia
    2. Resting tremor (Parkinson-like)
    3. Motor restlessness
    4. Amphetamine-like psychosis

69. _______ Which of the following are <u>sigma</u> opioid receptor agonists?

    1. Pentazocine
    2. Phencyclidine
    3. Cyclazocine
    4. Codeine

70. _______ Which of the following have convulsant metabolites?

    1. Analeridine
    2. Alphaprodine
    3. Meperidine
    4. Methadone

71. _______ Which of the following are opioid receptor agonists?

    1. Capsacin
    2. Endorphin
    3. Substance P
    4. Methionine enkephalin

<u>MULTIPLE TRUE - FALSE</u>
<u>Directions Summarized:</u>

1	2	3	4	5
1,2,3	1,3	2,4	4	all are
only	only	only	only	correct

72. _______ Tolerance to the effects of morphine:

1. Develops equally to all of morphine's effects
2. Results in the development of cross-tolerance to oxycodone
3. Is not a significant factor in clinical practice
4. Is due to a change in neuronal sensitivity to the narcotic

73. _______ Constipation induced by narcotics:

1. Is induced by activation of narcotic receptors in the GI tract
2. Results in relaxation of the longitudinal smooth muscles
3. Occurs with codeine
4. Can occur with diphenoxylate without CNS effects

74. _______ Local anesthetic agents:

1. Prevent the generation of the nerve action potential
2. Block the potassium channel
3. Prevent the propagation of the nerve impulse
4. Act by binding calcium within the nerve membrane

75. _______ Phencyclidine overdose:

1. May result in coma
2. Can be treated with gastric lavage and acidification of the urine
3. Can result in violent behavior
4. Can be totally reversed with i.v. naloxone

76. _______ Following acute injection morphine may produce:

1. Nausea and vomiting
2. Biliary colic
3. Itching due to histamine release
4. Sedation leading to sleep

<u>MATCHING</u>

      1. Naloxone
      2. Buprenorphine
      3. Both
      4. Neither

77. _______ Produces analgesia and sedation
78. _______ Antagonist in narcotic addicts
79. _______ Will reverse the depressant effects of Pentazocine

* * * * * * * * * *

      1. Nitrous oxide
      2. Halothane
      3. Both
      4. Neither

80. _______ Analgesia
81. _______ Hypotension

* * * * * * * * * *

      1. Phenobarbital
      2. Diazepam
      3. Both
      4. Neither

82. _______ Has a potential for withdrawal symptoms which include convulsions and toxic psychosis
83. _______ Has pharmacologically active metabolites
84. _______ Produces clinically important microsomal enzyme induction

* * * * * * * * * *

      1. LSD
      2. Psilocin
      3. Mescaline
      4. Phencyclidine
      5. THC

85. _______ Most potent; visual disturbances are most pronounced effect
86. _______ Conjunctival reddening; mood intensifier; euphoria state includes easy laughter, time and space perception alterations
87. _______ Once marketed as an anesthetic; a combative, hostile, antisocial state can occur
88. _______ A period of nausea, tremor, and perspiration precedes the LSD-like dream state

ANSWERS

1. ___3___ Diarrhea. The narcotic analgesic drugs cause constipation. The original medical use of opium was for relief of diarrhea and dysentery. They are still the most effective agents. Remember little tolerance develops to constipation and miotic effect.

2. ___3___ Potency. These compounds are very similar in their actions. An effective dose of LSD is 25 μg, psilocybin 4 **mg**, and mescaline 0.2 **g**.

3. ___2___ Sedation. The sedation with increasing doses of antianxiety drugs progress to anaesthesia and coma. The sedation with antipsychotics is more of a state of indifference or apathy, with a drowsy feeling and motor inactivity, but they can be aroused. Antianxiety drugs, but not antipsychotics, produce physical dependence (similar to barbiturates) and muscle-relaxant activity; antipsychotics produce extrapyramidal symptoms, tremors and spastic movements, and some of the phenothiazines are potent antiemetics.

4. ___1___ The central depressant actions of the barbiturates are terminated by three mechanisms: very short acting-very lipid soluble compounds, by physical redistribution; short and intermediate acting compounds, such as pentobarbital, by metabolism--generally to a hydroxylated compound, and long acting-low lipid soluble compounds, by renal excretion as well as metabolism.

5. ___4___ High blood levels of the local anesthetic agents can occur. Problems are generally for this cause.

6. ___4___

7. ___3___ This is the distinguishing difference between enflurane and the other anesthetic agents and is the reason this anesthetic is not used in patients with seizure foci.

8. ___4___

9. ___4___ MPTP was a byproduct in the illicit manufacturer of meperidine-like compounds. MPTP is a protoxin taken up by astrocytes and metabolized by MAO to a stable charged ion that selectively damages striatal dopaminergic neurons. Ecstasy (MDMA) is reported in animals to destroy serotoninergic neurons.

10. ___4___ Freon is a group of halogenated hydrocarbons containing one or more fluorine moieties. Potential of catecholamine-induced cardiac arrhythmias is a potential for any halogenated hydrocarbon. Selected populations abuse various solvents including gasoline, paint and glue.

11. ___3___

12. ___5___ Analgesic efficacy for aspirin and acetaminophen are equal. Since both work by inhibition of cyclooxygenase (prostaglandin synthetase) there is no increase in efficacy with the combination. Additive efficacy occurs with codeine and either aspirin or acetaminophen because of different mechanisms of action.

13. ___4___

14. ___4___ Ethanol and other sedative-hypnotics have excitatory effects caused by depression of inhibitory pathways from the cortex (i.e., a loss of inhibition rather than a direct stimulation).

15. ___4___

16. ___4___

17. ___4___ Caffeine is more potent for CNS stimulation.

18.   3   More complications have occurred with too vigorous treatment. While the non-effectiveness of general CNS stimulants has been known for a long time, once the patient reaches the hospital most of the complications in barbiturate overdose have resulted from hypernatremia by using sodium bicarbonate for urinary alkalinization, and fluid overload and pulmonary edema from either hemodialysis or hemoperfusion.

19.   5

20.   4

21.   4

22.   2

23.   5   Triazolam is marketed exclusively as a hypnotic while alprazolam is marketed for anxiety, particularly with depression.

24.   4   Malnutrition. Remember that malnutrition is not only caused by inadequate dietary intake but also by GI absorption impairment, pancreatic insufficiently, defective cofactors for metabolism, and storage of nutrients.

25.   4

26.   3

27.   2   Morphine, methadone, and codeine are <u>mu</u> and <u>kappa</u> agonists, while <u>butorphanol</u>, a mixed agonist-antagonist works through the <u>sigma</u> and <u>kappa</u> receptor. The increase in blood pressure, heart rate and pulmonary artery pressure are <u>sigma effects</u> as well as dysphoria and hallucinations which may be observed.

28.   4

29.   4   MAC is an abbreviation for the minimum alveolar concentration [a dose] that will prevent movement caused by surgical incision in 50% of the patients.

30.   3   Saturation of metabolic pathways occur in the therapeutic range, so phenytoin follows Michaelis-Menten kinetics rather than first order or zero order kinetics. Thus, therapeutic monitoring of phenytoin blood levels is required because there is a substantial interindividual variation between dose and resulting blood concentration.

31.   5   Tolerance develops rather rapidly to the anticonvulsant actions of benzodiazepines in contrast to the barbiturates. This limits their prophylactic use in epilepsy.

32.   3   Alkaline urine will increase the amount of the ionized form of the drug (pKa 3.5). This form will be excreted; the unionized form available for reabsorption through the tubules will be decreased in an alkaline urine. The pKs of the other compounds are such that alkalinzation of urine will have little effect on excretion.

33.   1

34.   2   Contrary to its use as a study aide, amphetamine has no ability to improve learning.

35.   3   Codeine is the only drug listed which selectively interacts with narcotic receptors.

36.   5   There is no difference in efficacy for the antidepressants. The choice of therapy depends on whether sedation is or is not desired and primarily on anticholinergic and cardiovascular side effects.

37.   1   Antipsychotic drugs rather than antidepressant drugs have Parkinsonian-like effects as one of their major adverse effects.

38.   2   Desipramine is an active metabolite of imipramine.

39.   2

40.   5

41.   3

42.   3   Naloxone will reverse the effects of pentazocine but requires high doses. Use of doxapram or caffeine as respiratory stimulants in this case is not rational. Caffeine is used to treat apnea particularly in the premature infant.

43.   1

44.   4   Nitrous oxide has a low Ostwald partition coefficient, 0.47 compared to 12 for ether. If nitrous oxide was more potent it probably would be the drug of choice for most surgical anesthesia. Both nitrous oxide and ether have strong analgesic properties (when compared to other general anesthetics, but not to morphine). Nitrous oxide has little effect on respiration and poor muscle relaxation properties.

45.   2   While tolerance will develop at a different rate for different narcotic analgesics, it always develops faster at higher doses with a frequent dosing schedule. Obviously if the dose is small enough and over an extended time period no tolerance will occur. Tolerance does not develop at the same rate for all actions. Little tolerance occurs to the constipating, miotic and cortex-spinal stimulating effects. Tolerance develops quickly to respiratory depression, tolerance develops slightly slower to the euphoria and analgesia. Cross tolerance exists between the narcotic analgesics. Disappearance of tolerance has a variable course but is similar to the changes in physical dependence which are progessively lost in withdrawal.

46.   1   Meperidine is a narcotic analgesic; secobarbital and alcohol are sedative-hypnotics. Both classes produce physical dependence and marked withdrawal. Withdrawal from the sedative-hypnotic class is often marked by convulsions which can be life threatening. Marihuana does not produce physical dependence; there are no consistent withdrawal signs or symptoms.

47.   1   Disulfiram inhibits dopamine-beta hydroxylase, xanthine oxidase and acetaldehyde dehydrogenase. It does not affect alcohol dehydrogenase, so after ethanol consumption, acetaldehyde accumulates, which produces flushing, vasodilation, decreased blood pressure, tachycardia, and vomiting. In extreme cases coma and even death have been reported.

48.   5   All of the agents listed can decrease the patients reaction to pain. Most studies show that a placebo is effective in 30-35% of the patients with mild to moderate pain.

49.   5

50.   1   Buspirone is a new anxiolytic agent that does not produce muscle relaxation, or have other properties of sedative-hypnotic drugs.

51.   5   Diazepam, to treat convulsions; O_2, to prevent hypoxia, decrease risk of convulsions; artificial respiration, if breathing is inadequate; i.v. fluids, if blood pressure drops; cardiovascular support drugs, if low BP persists and/or heart rate drops.

52.   2   The use of epinephrine delays systemic absorption; as a result, duration of action is longer and blood concentrations are lower (toxicity reduced).

53.   2   Sleep walking with complex and, at times, violent behavior is treated with phenytoin or carbamazepine. Primary enuresis is treated initially with behavioral therapy and if necessary, with imipramine.

54.   5

55.   2   Treatment is the same as for Parkinson's disease. Chlorpromazine and haloperidol are dopamine blockers.

56. __2__
57. __5__
58. __3__ Although flurazepam is rapidly metabolized, its active metabolite has a long half life and action.
59. __2__
60. __3__
61. __4__
62. __2__ All four drugs are used as anesthetic induction agents. For the high risk patients etomidate and midazolam are considered better choices because transient decreases in blood pressure, respiratory depression, laryngospasm or bronchospasm are less likely to occur.
63. __3__
64. __2__
65. __1__
66. __1__
67. __4__
68. __1__
69. __1__ Recent studies has established that phencyclidine binds to the _sigma_ opiate receptor, which accounts for part of its effects. Codeine binds to the _mu_ receptor.
70. __2__
71. __3__
72. __3__
73. __5__
74. __2__
75. __1__
76. __5__
77. __2__
78. __3__
79. __1__
80. __1__
81. __2__
82. __3__
83. __2__
84. __1__
85. __1__
86. __5__
87. __4__
88. __3__

AUTACOIDS

I. <u>HISTAMINE AND ITS ANTAGONISTS</u>

   A. <u>HISTAMINE</u>
     1. General Considerations:
       a. Tissue localization:
         1) Endogenous amine found in blood, purulent exudate, gastric juice, platelets, leukocytes and many tissues in the body.
         2) Particularly prominent in the skin, GI tract and the lung.
         3) Bound to heparin in the mast cells in tissues and basophils in blood.
       b. Biosynthesis and metabolism:
         1) Derived from the amino acid histidine by histidine decarboxylase in all tissues in which it is found; also formed by bacteria in the GI tract.
         2) Metabolized by methylation before being oxidized by monoamine oxidase.
       c. Tissue release:
         1) Released and production stimulated by damage to cells and tissues.
         2) Also can be liberated from tissue stores by histamine liberators (48/80) plus snake venoms and drugs such as curare, morphine and others.
         3) Antigen-antibody reactions.
     2. Pharmacologic Actions:
       a. Cardiovascular:
         1) Parenteral administration in human results in capillary dilation, decreased venous return, reduction in blood pressure and cardiac output.
         2) Hypotension is of short duration due to rapid metabolism of histamine and compensatory release of adrenal catecholamines.
       b. Smooth muscle:
         1) Vascular smooth muscle relaxed; most other smooth muscle contracted.
         2) Stimulatory (constrictor) effects most prominent on the uterus and bronchi; less prominent on the GI tract and least prominent on the urinary bladder and gallbladder.
       c. Glands: Stimulated secretions from the salivary, bronchial and gastric glands, among others.
       d. Miscellaneous:
         1) Release of catecholamines from the adrenal medulla
         2) A chemical mediator of pain and itch
         3) May be one of the chemical mediators of anaphylactic shock (the signs and symptoms of systemic anaphylaxis very closely resemble those of the parenteral administration of histamine).
     3. Toxicity:
       a. Most prominent life-threatening symptoms are shock (general vasodilation, marked fall in blood pressue) and severe bronchoconstriction.
       b. Most prominent effects, therefore, are on smooth muscle

    c. Most effective physiologic antagonist is epinephrine; antihistamines are not particularly effective in severe toxicity

4. Therapeutic Uses: None at the present time
Has been employed in the diagnosis of: achlorhydria (inability of histamine to induce gastric secretions) and pheochromocytoma (histamine-induced release of adrenal catecholamines).

5. Receptor Type:
H_1 receptor subserves most effects; gastric acid secretion is subserved by the H_2 receptor type.

B. <u>H_1-BLOCKING AGENTS (ANTIHISTAMINES)</u>:
1. Drugs which antagonize some of the pharmacologic actions of histamine (those subserved by the H_1 type receptor); in addition, they possessing sedative, local anesthetic, anticholinergic, adrenergic and antispasmodic properties.

2. General Considerations:
    a. Contain the ethylamine structure in common with acetylcholine, histamine, adrenergic agents, and local anesthetics
    b. Well absorbed orally and parenterally

3. Mechanism of Action:
    a. Classified as competitive antagonists of the Histamine – 1 receptor
    b. Differential histamine receptor antagonism: edema and itch (good); hypotension (poor); gastric secretion – none; this function subserved by the H_2 receptor, not the H_1 receptor, and is not affected by classic drugs.

4. Pharmacologic Actions:
    a. CNS:
        1) Many posess sedative properties; this is the rationale for their use in over-the counter "sleeping" preparations.
        2) May induce CNS stimulation
        3) Some posess antiemetic effects
        4) Some are effective against motion sickness
    b. Autonomic System: many possess anticholinergic properties
    c. Allergy
        1) Do not prevent the release of histamine from mast cells by Ag-Ab union
        2) Pre-treatment with the antihistamines does not prevent the signs and symptoms of allergy not mediated by histamine
        3) Antihistamines merely modify some of the signs and symptoms of histamine release (edema, itching)
    d. Miscellaneous: Most have local anesthetic and quinidine-like properties

5. Toxicity:
    a. Side effects (generally possess a high therapeutic index):
        1) Sedation (most common)
        2) GI: nausea and vomiting, anorexia, diarrhea, stomach upset, constipation
        3) Headache, faintness, visual disturbance, hypotension
    b. Acute toxicity:
        1) Adults: usually CNS depression and coma
        2) Children: usually CNS stimulation (excitement, hallucinations, convulsions) followed by CNS depression

6. Therapeutic Uses and Selected Agents:
    a. Allergy (to relieve itching and edema) and allergic rhinitis:

          1) Tripelennamine
          2) Diphenhydramine
          3) Chlorpheniramine
          4) <u>Terfenadine</u>: A new H_1-receptor blocking agent: appears to not cause sedation; chemically different from classic agents.
      b. Emesis and motion sickness
          1) Dimenhydrinate
          2) Cyclizine

C. <u>H_2-BLOCKING AGENTS</u>
1. Recently developed agents which specifically antagonize the actions of histamine on the H_2 receptor; competitive blockade produced.
2. Some effects of histamine which are difficult to block with classic H_1 receptor antagonists (e.g., vasodilator actions) can be antagonized by a combination of a classic H_1 antihistaminic agent plus a new H_2 receptor antagonist.
3. Agents:
   a. <u>Cimetidine</u>: Inhibits gastric secretion caused by histamine, gastrin, ACh or food; well absorbed; adverse effects are rare—antiandrogenic effect in large doses may cause gynecomastia in men (reversible) and galactorrhea in women; slurred speech and disorientation may occur in elderly; blood dyscrasias are rare. Inhibits hepatic drug metabolizing enzymes and may potentiate other drugs also metabolized by this system.
   b. <u>Ranitidine</u>: Greater potency and longer duration of action; does not inhibit hepatic drug metabolizing enzymes; no antiandrogenic effect.
4. Effective in treatment of duodenal ulcer, Zollinger-Ellison syndrome, and reflux esophagitis.

D. <u>CROMOLYN SODIUM</u>
Inhibits the release of histamine and other autacoids from mast cells in the lung; used for prophylaxis of asthma.

II. <u>SEROTONIN AND ITS ANTAGONISTS</u>

A. <u>SEROTONIN (5-Hydroxytryptamine)</u>
1. General Consideration:
   a. Tissue localization:
      1) Endogenous amine present in large amounts in the enterochromaffin system of the intestine and in platelets, where its function is unknown.
      2) Presence in brain has led to speculation that it functions there as a central neurotransmitter.
      3) Synthesized from tryptophan; degraded by monoamine oxidase to form 5-hydroxy indoleacetic acid (5-HIAA), metabolic product excreted in urine; 5-HIAA excretion will increase greatly in the presence of a carcinoid tumor; ingestion of bananas increases excretion of 5-HIAA since bananas contain large amounts of serotonin.
2. Pharmacologic Actions:
   a. Cardiovascular: Intravenous injection of a few micrograms produces a triphasic response, 1) a transient fall in blood

pressure. 2) brief hypertension, and 3) prolonged hypotension (direct and reflex effects).
    b. Respiratory system: I.V. injection, initial apnea followed by hyperpnea.
    c. Smooth muscle:
        1) GI muscle contracts; direct effect and because ganglion cells stimulated
        2) Bronchial smooth muscle constricts
    d. Miscellaneous:
        1) Serotonin can stimulate efferent nerve endings, ganglion cells, and adrenal medullary cells
        2) Considerable speculation about role of serotonin in CNS - relationship to hallucinogenic drugs, etc.
        3) Serotonin is responsible for some of the symptoms of the <u>carcinoid syndrome</u>; these tumors may contain and release serotonin, bradykinin (kinin-producing enzymes), epinephrine and histamine among other things. Effects seen are: 1) flushing - due to arteriolar dilatation, 2) wide swings in blood pressure - due to direct vasoconstrictor and indirect vasodilator actions, 3) colic - intense cramping of GI tract from constrictor effect, and 4) bronchiolar constriction.

B. <u>SEROTONIN ANTAGONISTS</u>
    Several pharmacologic antagonists of serotonin have important therapeutic applications which have nothing to do with an anti-serotonin action. Serotonin antagonists include numerous lysergic acid derivatives, many of which are naturally occurring ergot alkaloids.

  1. <u>Methysergide</u> - potent antiserotonin clinically useful in treatment of migraine headache and carcinoid syndrome.
  2. <u>Chlorpromazine</u> - many antihistamine and <u>alpha</u> adrenergic blocking drugs also block the effects of serotonin.
  3. <u>Cyproheptadine</u> - potent antihistamine and antiserotonin, clinically useful in treatment of pruritic dermatoses and carcinoid syndrome.

VASOACTIVE PEPTIDES

A variety of naturally occurring vasoactive polypeptides have been described. Some of these agents and their prominent actions are:

A. <u>BRADYKININ</u>
  1. Formed from <u>alpha</u>$_2$ globulin precursor, bradykininogen, by the plasma enzyme kallikrein; in body tissues, the glandular enzyme, kallikrein, converts kallidinogen to kallidin (lys - bradykinin); kallidin then transformed in tissues to bradykinin. Bradykinin is inactivated by kininase I (carboxypeptidase) and kininase II (angiotensin converting enzyme).
  2. Bradykinin is a marked vasodilator; 50x potency of histamine as a dilator, which itself is quite potent.
  3. Bradykinin also is a potent constrictor of GI smooth muscle, bronchioles, and uterine smooth muscle; increases capillary permeability and causes pain.

4. Releases catecholamines from the adrenal medulla; catecholamine release, along with vasodilation-induced reflex activation, causes an increase in cardiac output.
5. Bradykinin is involved in the carcinoid syndrome: tumor of argentachromaffin cells of the gut which produce large amounts of amines, bradykinin, histamine and serotonin. Patient will become flushed, have wide swings in blood pressure, develop diarrhea due to gut-stimulating effects of these agents, wheeze due to bronchiolar stimulation and constriction, develop intense migrane-like headaches caused by dilation and edema of cerebral blood vessels. Headache of cardinoid syndrome is blocked by aspirin and other anti-inflammatory agents. Migrane is not affected by aspirin.
6. The kallikrein-kinin system is an intrinsic part of the blood coagulation mechanism.

B. ANGIOTENSIN
1. The enzyme, renin, acts on precursor plasma $alpha_2$ globulin, angiotensinogen, to form angiotensin I (which has little activity); in the lung (primarily) angiotensin I is converted to angiotensin II by the enzyme, dipeptide hydrolase (converting enzyme); angiotensin II is degraded by angiotensinase to inactive peptides. Conversion of angiotensin I to II is limited in the plasma; major conversion occurs in the lung.
2. Angiotensin II constricts arteriolar smooth muscle to give a pressor effect; very potent agent.
3. Stimulates the zona glomerulosa of the adrenal cortex to release aldosterone; stimulates the adrenal medulla to release catecholamines, which also contributes to vascular effects.
4. The renin-angiotensin system has been implicated in certain forms of hypertension.
5. Converting enzyme inhibitors (captopril, enalapril) and receptor antagonist (saralasin) are available for diagnostic use (renovascular disease) and as antihypertensive drugs. Coverting enzyme inhibitors also are useful to treat congestive heart failure.

PROSTAGLANDINS (and related agents)

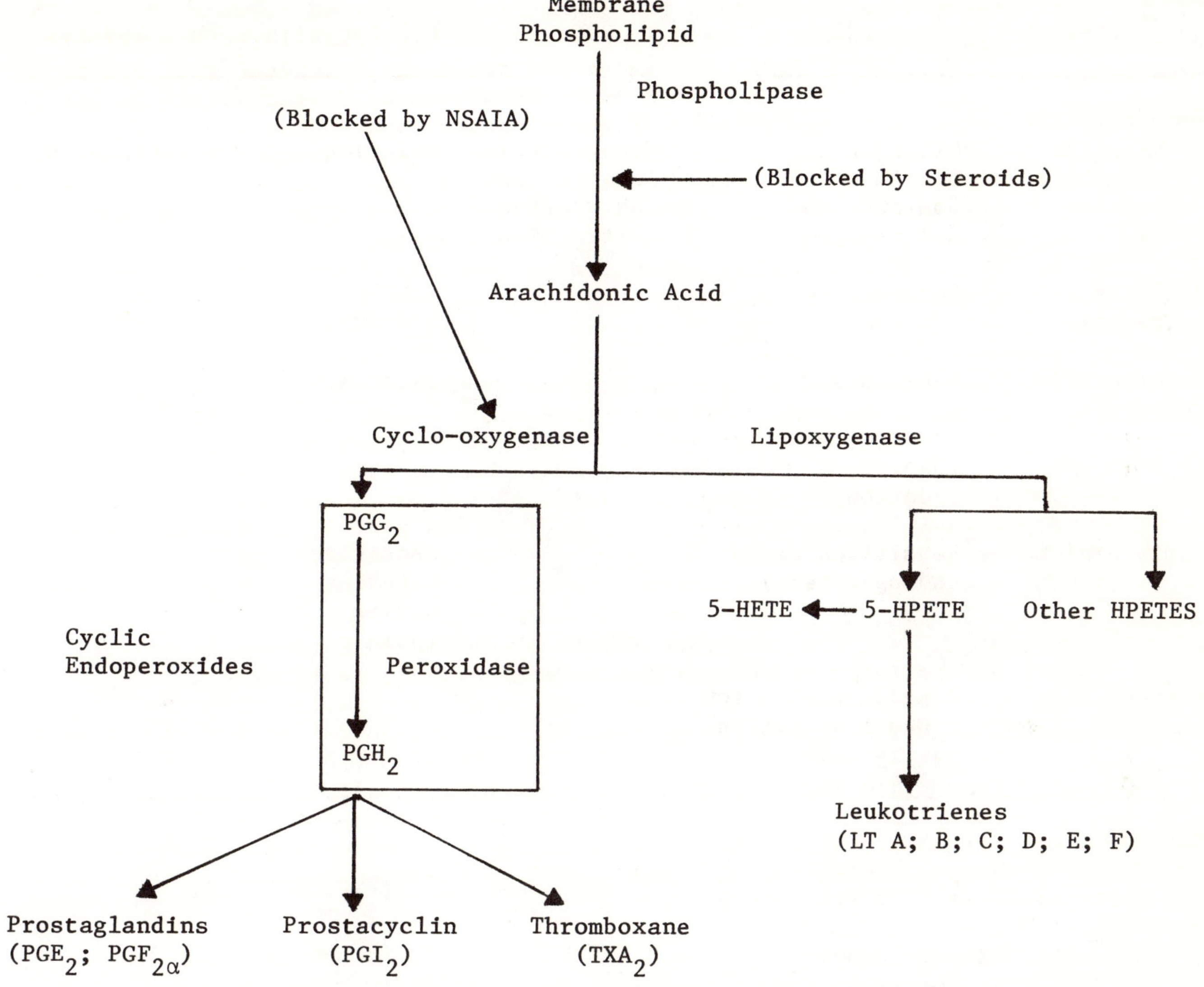

A family of endogenous lipid substances, rapidly synthesized and degraded (in pulmonary, renal and hepatic vascular beds) and having widespread occurrence in tissues. Speculation is that they play an important regulatory role on a variety of body functions, possibly also in a variety of clinical conditions. Major effects are exerted on the uterus, cardiovascular system, bronchi, GI tract, platelets, nervous system, and inflammatory and immune mechanisms. Aspirin and other non-steroidal anti-inflammatory agents (NSAIA) block the synthesis of prostaglandins; these agents may exert their effects through the inhibition of cyclo-oxygenase, preventing the formation of PGG_2 and H_2 which are the immediate precursors of all other prostaglandins. Lipoxygenase products are involved mainly with cell mediated mechanisms and have important functions in immune responses. These products are not reduced by aspirin-like drugs.

Some Important Actions of PGs, Prostacyclin and Thromboxanes

System	PGEs	PGFs	Prostacyclin	Thromboxanes
Smooth muscle:				
Vascular	Dilation	Constriction	Dilation	Constriction
Bronchial	Dilation	Constriction		
Uterine	Contraction	Contraction		
GI	Contraction	Contraction		
Platelet aggregation	Inhibits ($\uparrow\Delta$ AMP)		Inhibits ($\uparrow\Delta$ AMP)	Stimulates ($\downarrow\Delta$ AMP)
Gastric Acid Secretion	Decreases		Decreases	
Central NS	Fever Sedation			
Peripheral NS	Sensitizes nerve endings (pain)		Sensitizes afferent nerves (pain)	
Kidney	$\uparrow$ Renal blood flow $\uparrow$ Renin secretion Natriuresis			

Therapeutics:

1. Abortificients (2nd trimester):

    a. PGE_2 (dinoprostone)
    b. $PGF_{2\alpha}$ (dinoprost)
    c. 15-methyl $PGF_{2\alpha}$ (carboprost tromethan)

2. Anti-ulcer – synthetic analog of PGE_1 (misoprostol)

NON-NARCOTIC ANALGESICS

Diverse group of drugs; not related to opiates; many are antipyretic analgesics; some have anti-inflammatory actions; some also useful in gout - uric acid blood levels are lowered. This group referred to as <u>nonsteroidal anti-inflammatory analgesics</u> (NSAIA).

I. <u>NSAIA</u>

These drugs which are analgesic, antipyretic and anti-inflammatory are thought to produce their effects by interfering with the production of prostaglandins (cyclo-oxygenase inhibition).

A. SALICYLATES

<u>Aspirin</u>: analgesic (not effective in severe or visceral pain), antipyretic, anti-inflammatory, and uricosuric (in <u>high</u> doses). Adverse effects: G.I. upset and hemorrhage, nausea and vomiting (irritates stomach and also acts on CTZ). Acid-base problems frequent (adults - usually see metabolic alkalosis probably due to increased respiration. In children usually see progression to metabolic acidosis). <u>Chronic intoxication</u>: "salicylism," headache, dizziness, tinnitus, nausea and vomiting. <u>Anti-inflammatory dose</u>: 4-10X higher than necessary for analgesia. Occult bleeding is a significant problem in the treatment of arthritis <u>Acute toxicity in children</u>: remove any unabsorbed drug by gastric lavage; treat acid-base problems; promote excretion by alkalinization of the urine; peritoneal or hemodialysis may be necessary. <u>Sodium salicylate</u>: Similar to aspirin, except more irritating to G.I. tract.

B. PROPIONIC ACID DERIVATIVES

<u>Ibuprofen</u>
<u>Naproxen</u>
<u>Fenoprofen</u>

Newly introduced group of compounds with analgesic, antipyretic, anti-inflammatory actions. Reported to have less G.I. toxicity than aspirin, but still fairly high incidence of G.I. effects and could exacerbate peptic ulcer; patients hypersensitive to aspirin also are hypersensitive to these compounds.

C. PYRAZOLONE DERIVATIVES

<u>Phenylbutazone</u>
<u>Oxyphenbutazone</u>
<u>Sulfinpyrazone</u>

Analgesic, antipyretic, anti-inflammatory and uricosuric. May cause blood dyscrasias, prolonged prothrombin time, G.I. upset. Phenylbutazone and congeners are classic examples of drugs that displace other drugs bound to plasma protein and as a result cause significant drug interaction toxicities. Because of the high incidence of blood dyscrasias, these compounds should be used for acute control of pain <u>only</u>.

D. ACETIC ACID DERIVATIVES

Indomethacin
Tolmetin
Sulindac (must be metabolized to an active form)

Analgesic, antipyretic and anti-inflammatory; G.I. problems, CNS
headache, hypersensitivity, blood dyscrasias, aplastic anemia;
contraindicated in children, pregnancy, hypersensitivity, and ulcer.

II. ANALGESIC-ANTIPYRETIC ONLY (not anti-inflammatory drugs)

ACETOPHENETIDIN (PHENACETIN)

ACETAMINOPHEN

Acetophenetidin (Phenacetin) and Acetaminophen are good analgesics and
antipyretics but have no anti-inflammatory or uricosuric actions.
Antipyretic and analgesic only. Is often sold as the "no aspirin" over the
counter analgesic. Due to the association of Reyes Syndrome in children
with aspirin use, acetaminophen is preferable in the treatment of fever in
children. Can substitute for aspirin for these effects but may be more
toxic. Parent compound acetophenetidin produces methemoglobinemia and
nephrotoxicity. Both may cause allergic reactions and hepatic necrosis.
Acetaminophen is associated with blood dyscrasias.

AGENTS USED IN GOUT

A. COLCHICINE

Used prophylactically and in acute gout. Not analgesic or
anti-inflammatory in itself. Prevents phagocytosis of uric acid
crystals by leukocytes, therefore blocks inflammatory response; side
effects include: nausea, vomiting, diarrhea and abdominal pain.

B. ALLOPURINOL

Used in treatment of chronic gout; inhibits xanthine oxidase, thus
reduces formation of uric acid. Well tolerated, may produce xanthine
renal stones. May precipitate acute attack at the start of therapy;
therefore, it is usually given with colchicine at the start.
Hypersensitivity is common toxicity.

C. PROBENECID AND SULFINPYRAZOL:

Increases urinary secretion of uric acid by preventing reuptake via
the renal tubular acid transport system. May be antagonized by
salicylates in early phase of treatment.

D. PHENYLBUTAZONE AND INDOMETHACIN

Effective in acute gout attacks and used in patients who do not
tolerate colchicine well.
Indomethacin now is the drug of choice for acute gout attacks.

OTHER AGENTS USED IN RHEUMATOID ARTHRITIS

A. GOLD SALTS

For injection only: gold thioglucose and gold thiomalate commonly
are used; probably most effective therapy; can arrest irreversible
damage; mechanism unknown; water-soluble, given i.m., accumulated in
inflamed tissue, slow renal excretion; high incidence of toxicity:
dermatitis with pruritus, stomatitis, toxic nephritis, hematological
depression (thrombocytopenia, aplastic anemia, agranulocytosis);
anaphylactoid reactions; contraindicated in systemic lupus, known
allergy and pregnancy.

ORALLY EFFECTIVE:

Auranofin: useful in the early management of arthritis. May cause GI
upset, diarrhea. Skin pigmentation due to effects of UV light or metal
in skin may occur.

B. CORTICOSTEROIDS

Often used when more traditional therapeutics does not show benefit.
Side effects limit aggressive use of these drugs. (See Hormones
Section).

C. HYDROXYCHLOROQUINE

Is preferred over chloroquine; given orally; beneficial effects
appear after several months; toxic reactions in 50% of patients (skin
eruptions, hair loss, nausea, vomiting, headache, neuromyopathy, visual
disturbances) usually are not serious and are reversible. However, an
infrequent irreversible retinopathy occurs, which must be weighed
against the probable, but modest benefits.

REVIEW QUESTIONS

<u>ONE BEST ANSWER</u>

1. _______ All of the following agents may contribute to the carcinoid syndrome EXCEPT:

    1. 5-Hydroxytryptamine (serotonin)
    2. Renin
    3. Histamine
    4. Bradykinin
    5. Epinephrine

2. _______ All of the following are true of bradykinin EXCEPT:

    1. Causes bronchodilation
    2. Is formed from plasma $\underline{alpha}_2$-globulin by kallikrein
    3. Causes pain upon subcutaneous injection
    4. Relaxes vascular smooth muscle
    5. Stimulates epinephrine secretion from the adrenal gland

3. _______ All of the following are true of angiotensin II EXCEPT:

    1. Stimulates the secretion of catecholamines
    2. Stimulates the secretion of aldosterone
    3. Increases peripheral vascular resistance
    4. Is activated by renin
    5. Is degraded by angiotensinase to inactive peptides

4. _______ The side effect common to most antihistaminic compounds in therapeutic doses is:

    1. Thrombocytopenia
    2. Insomnia
    3. Convulsions
    4. Achlorhydria
    5. Drowsiness

5. _______ All of the following conditions are <u>contraindications</u> to the use of acetylsalicylic acid for the treatment of rheumatoid arthritis EXCEPT:

    1. Hypertension
    2. Vitamin K deficiency
    3. Hypersensitivity
    4. Gastric ulcer
    5. Meniere's disease

<u>ONE BEST ANSWER</u>

6. _______ All of the following signs and symptoms may be associated with acute salicylate intoxication EXCEPT:

    1. Kussmaul respiration
    2. Gastrointestinal symptoms
    3. Petechial hemorrahages
    4. Hypothermia
    5. Acid-base balance disturbances

7. _______ One of the following is the drug of choice in relieving the pain of acute gout attacks:

    1. Indomethacin
    2. Gold thioglucose
    3. Allopurinol
    4. Probenecid
    5. Hydroxychloroquine

8. _______ Which of the following drugs inhibits uric acid excretion by inhibiting xanthine oxidase?

    1. Phenylbutazone
    2. Probenecid
    3. Allopurinol
    4. Colchicine
    5. Alpha tocopherol

9. _______ All of the following have significant anti-inflammatory actions EXCEPT:

    1. Acetaminophen
    2. Aspirin
    3. Indomethacin
    4. Phenylbutazone
    5. Sodium salicylate

10. _______ The <u>initial</u> disturbance in acute intoxication by salicylates is:

    1. Respiratory depression causing retention of CO_2
    2. Renal loss of fixed cation
    3. Respiratory stimulation causing loss of CO_2
    4. Inhibition of renal carbonic anhydrase
    5. Depression of the brain-stem reticular activating system

<u>ONE BEST ANSWER</u>

11. _______ Which one of the following prostaglandins or prostaglandin analogs is used clinically to inhibit gastric acid secretion?

1. Dinoprostone
2. Dinoprost
3. Misoprostol
4. Cytoprostol tromethamine
5. Carboprost tromethamine

12. _______ Which one of the following is an orally effective antiarthritic formulation?

1. Gold sodium malate
2. Aurothioglucose
3. Gold cyanide
4. Auranofin

13. _______ Increased uric acid elimination in the urine for the long term treatment of gout is best accomplished with:

1. Probenecid
2. Alkalinization of the urine to pH 12.0
3. Phenylbutazone
4. Acidification of the urine to pH 4.0

14. _______ Which one of the following is a pharmacologically inactive pro-drug?

1. Sulindac
2. Ibuprofen
3. Indomethacin
4. Fentanyl

15. _______ All of the following are true of prostaglandins <u>EXCEPT</u>:

1. Are 20 carbon fatty acids
2. Are hormones
3. Are inactivated by 15-OH-PG dehydrogenase
4. Are vasoactive agents
5. Are derived from arachidonic acid

<u>MULTIPLE TRUE-FALSE</u>
Directions: For each of the statements below, <u>ONE</u> or <u>MORE</u> of the completions given is correct.

> 1 - If only 1, 2 and 3 are correct
> 2 - If only 1 and 3 are correct
> 3 - If only 2 and 4 are correct
> 4 - If only 4 is correct
> 5 - If all are correct

16. _______ Histamine in man can:

1. Cause a reflex tachycardia
2. Be released during an antigen-antibody response
3. Increase the output of gastric acid
4. Cause release of catecholamines from a pheochromocytoma

17. _______ Antihistamines such as diphenhydramine can:

1. Reduce the fall in blood pressure caused by histamine
2. Block the secretion of gastric acid evoked by histamine
3. Reduce the bronchoconstriction caused by histamine
4. Prevent the release of histamine from mast cells

18. _______ Renin:

1. Is a potent vasoconstrictor
2. Is released by sympathetic nerve activation
3. Converts angiotensin I to angiotensin II
4. Release is stimulated by low blood volume

19. _______ Captropril:

1. Is orally effective
2. May lower blood pressure in patients with "normal" renin levels
3. Decreases the circulating amount of angiotensin II
4. Inhibits enzymes that inactivate bradykinin

20. _______ Angiotensin II:

1. Blocks autonomic ganglia
2. Acts in CNS to promote thirst
3. Inhibits secretion of antidiuretic hormone (ADH)
4. Is a more potent vasoconstrictor than is norepinephrine

21. _______ Bradykinin:

1. Is inactivated by the same enzyme that activates angiotensin I
2. Is a potent vasodilator
3. May contract smooth muscle of the gut
4. Is destroyed by passage through the pulmonary circulation

<u>MULTIPLE TRUE - FALSE</u>
<u>Directions Summarized:</u>

1	2	3	4	5
1,2,3	1,3	2,4	4	all are
only	only	only	only	correct

22. _______ Which of the following are common side effects of antihistamine therapy with H_1-blockers?

1. Sedation
2. Dryness of the mouth
3. Nausea, vomiting and epigastric distress
4. Agranulocytosis

23. _______ Which of the following are effectively antagonized by H_1-blocking drugs?

1. Allergic bronchoconstriction
2. Gastric acid secretion
3. Release of histamine from mast cells
4. Hay fever symptoms

24. _______ Serotonin produces which of the following effects?

1. Decreases in blood pressure in humans
2. Stimulation of sensory nerve endings
3. Increased gut motility
4. Disturbance of the electrical properties of the heart

25. _______ Inhibition of cyclo-oxygenase might be expected to:

1. Inhibit prostacyclin synthesis
2. Inhibit thromboxane synthesis
3. Increase leukotriene levels
4. Cause pregnancy

26. _______ Which of the following are true with regard to thromboxane A_2?

1. Inhibits platelet aggregation
2. Increases platelet cyclic AMP levels
3. Produces vasodilation of blood vessels
4. Induces platelet aggregation

27. _______ Aspirin is used in the treatment of:

1. Inflammation
2. Hypothermia
3. Pain
4. Morphine withdrawal

<u>MULTIPLE TRUE – FALSE</u>
Directions Summarized:

1	2	3	4	5
1,2,3 only	1,3 only	2,4 only	4 only	all are correct

28. ______ Which of the following produce therapeutic effects by interfering with prostaglandin synthesis?

    1. Acetaminophen
    2. Auranofin
    3. Indomethacin
    4. Lithium

29. ______ Inhibition of prostaglandin synthesis by aspirin is associated with which of the following effects?

    1. Antipyresis
    2. Anti-inflammatory
    3. Analgesia
    4. Antianxiety

<u>MATCHING</u>

Match the drugs with their <u>principle</u> uses

    1. Cimetidine
    2. Chlorpheniramine
    3. Cromolyn
    4. Cyclizine
    5. Cyproheptadine

30. ______ Prevention of motion sickness

31. ______ Treatment of carcinoid

32. ______ Treatment of allergic symptoms when drowsiness must be avoided

33. ______ Treatment of peptic ulcer

34. ______ Prophylactic treatment of bronchial asthma

<u>MATCHING</u>

Match the drug with the therapeutic use and toxicity

1. Acetaminophen
2. Aspirin
3. Phenylbutazone
4. Indomethacin
5. Ibuprofen

35. _______ Acute gout; aplastic anemia; agranulocytosis

36. _______ Antiinflammatory; analgesic; antipyretic; occult bleeding rare

37. _______ Closes ductus arteriosus; severe frontal headache common with chronic use

* * * * * * * * * *

1. Aspirin
2. Acetaminophen
3. Both
4. Neither

38. _______ Treatment of rheumatic fever

39. _______ Hepatic toxicity on overdose, treat with N-acetylcysteine

40. _______ Prevents platelet aggregation

ANSWERS

1.   2

2.   1

3.   4   Renin acts to produce angiotensin I.

4.   5

5.   1   Aspirin will worsen all of the listed conditions <u>except hypertension</u>. Aspirin-induced tinnitus and hearing loss are due to increased labyrinthine pressure, as is the case with Meniere's disease. As with vitamin K deficiency, aspirin will decrease prothrombin and cause hemorrhagic phenomena, and thus should be avoided in patients with ulcers. Hypersensitivity to aspirin usually involves skin rashes or anaphylaxis.

6.   4   The correct response is <u>hypothermia</u>. Aspirin will not lower the temperature of an afebrile patient and can cause hyperthermia at toxic plasma levels.

7.   1   <u>Indomethacin</u> is the agent of choice in relieving the pain of acute gout attacks. Allopurinol or probenecid are useful in the therapy of chronic gout but are contraindicated in acute attacks. Hydroxychloroquine and gold salts are used in other arthritic conditions.

8.   3   Xanthine oxidase is inhibited by <u>allopurinol</u>. This drug is a prime example of a compound synthesized for theoretical reasons, which has proved useful.

9.   1   <u>Acetaminophen</u> (and aminophenols in general) lack anti-inflammatory effects.

10.   3   The correct response is <u>respiratory stimulation causing loss of CO_2</u>, which is the initial disturbance in acute salicylate intoxication. Salicylates stimulate respiration directly and indirectly, but stimulation of medullary respiratory centers is the dominant effect in acute poisoning. Hyperpnea results in a fall in plasma pCO_2.

11.   3

12.   4

13.   1

14.   1

15.   2

16.   5

17.   2   Remember that there are specific H_1 and H_2 blockers with specific physiological effects.

18.   3

19.   5

20.   3

21.   5

22.   1

23.   4

24.   1

25.   1   33.   1

26.   4   34.   3

27.   2   35.   3

28.   2   36.   5

29.   1   37.   4

30.   4   38.   1

31.   5   39.   2

32.   2   40.   1

DIURETIC AGENTS

Diuretic drugs, agents which increase the volume of urine and promote the net loss of solute (NaCl) and water, are useful in treating a variety of diseases associated with edema formation (abnormal retention of salt and water by the kidney), especially congestive heart failure and cirrhosis of the liver. Some of these agents also have efficacy in the treatment of several non-edematous conditions such as essential hypertension.

Diuretic drugs must be used judiciously and their mechanism of action clearly understood, for numerous electrolyte abnormalities may follow their administration. The most serious is hypokalemia. Patients receiving digitalis and diuretics, for example, may develop severe cardiac arrhythmias precipitated by the reduction in serum potassium. Patients on lithium therapy may experience lithium toxicity after vigorous or prolonged diuretic therapy.

A. **THIAZIDES:** **Hydrochlorothiazide is the prototype**

Benzothiadiazide or thiazides are organic sulfonamide derivatives discovered during studies on carbonic anhydrase inhibitors. **Thiazides differ only in potency, bioavailability, and duration of action.** After oral administration – duration about 6-12 hours; given i.v. the duration is about 2-4 hours. **All produce same degree of diuresis with equipotent doses** (same efficacy).

Actions

Act primarily at distal tubule (cortical diluting site) – **decreased reabsorption of Na^+ with Cl^-** and H_2O reabsorption also decreased; **K+ secreted** (amount of sodium delivered or present in distal tubule is one of the determinants of potassium secretion – thiazides inhibit Na^+ reabsorption and thus augment K^+ secretion); **get increased urinary excretion of sodium, chloride and potassium, increased urine volume and slight alkalosis.** Most thiazides retain **weak carbonic anhydrase activity** – this effect may result in slight increase in bicarbonate excretion with alkaline urine (dose dependent).

Systemically the effect of potassium depletion to cause alkalosis is more important over the tendency towards acidosis from bicarbonate loss. Thus, with large doses, thiazides can cause **hypokalemic alkalosis.**

Although acid – base balance does not profoundly affect diuresis, with large doses **hypovolemia** may be induced with resulting loss of effectiveness of further thiazide therapy.

Clinical Uses:

Fluid Retention States: Edema of congestive heart failure, nephrotic edema, cirrhosis, retention of sodium caused by steroid therapy, etc.
Essential Hypertension: Thiazide compounds reduce blood pressure in hypertensive subjects – to a much lesser extent in normals – mechanism unknown.
Hypercalciuria: Acts on tubules to decrease excretion of calcium thus is useful in patients with calcium nephrolithiasis.
Diabetes insipidus: Urine output reduced in both types of diabetes insipidus (ADH sensitive and ADH insensitive).

<u>Adverse Effects:</u>

<u>Side effects</u> - weakness, fatigue, paresthesias, GI disturbances, skin rash, blood dyscrasias, photosensitivity and other hypersensitivity reactions

<u>Dose related toxicity:</u>

<u>Hypokalemia</u> - potassium depletion symptoms (neurological, muscle); may precipitate arrhythmias in digitalis treated patients

<u>Hypomagnesemia</u> - also may precipitate arrhythmias in digitalized patients

<u>Mild hyperglycemia</u> (impaired glucose tolerance) - probably due to decreased insulin secretion caused by hypokalemia

<u>Hyperuricemia</u> - thiazides are weak acids, secreted by proximal tubules and interfere with uric acid secretion by these cells - can precipitate gouty arthritis in susceptible patients.

<u>Decreased renal excretion of ammonia</u> - if alkaline urine from bicarbonate excretion - H+ secretion decreased and ammonia retained.

<u>Triglycerides and plasma cholesterol levels</u> - may be increased with antihypertensive therapy.

<u>Related (Thiazide-like) Agents</u>

<u>Chlorthalidone</u>

A sulfonamide but non-thiazide derivative - pharmacologically behaves like a thiazide, however. Same actions, same side effects, but longer duration of action - 2 to 3 days.

B. <u>HIGH-CEILING OR LOOP DIURETICS:</u>

<u>Maximal diuretic effect</u> is much greater than that seen with other diuretics.

1. <u>Furosemide is the prototype</u>

A sulfonamide derivative and retains some of the properties of thiazides; a weak inhibitor of carbonic anhydrase. Rapid onset of action after oral administration; short duration (4 hours); high degree of binding to plasma proteins and can displace other drugs such as warfarin.

<u>Actions</u>

Acts primarily on <u>ascending limb of the loop of Henle</u> to inhibit active reabsorption of chloride. Also has effect on renal vasculature to increase blood flow in the <u>vasa recta</u> - redistributes blood flow to cortical nephrons where less sodium reabsorption occurs. Get <u>increased excretion of Na^+, Cl^-, K^+ and NH_4^+, marked increase of urine volume</u> (get effective diuretic effect even in dehydrated patient with hypovolemia); Ca^{2+} and Mg^{2+} excretion also increased by furosemide.

<u>Can get hypochloremic, hypokalemic alkalosis</u>; "Contraction alkalosis" - large loss of water along with sodium and chloride, but not bicarbonate - get "contraction" of ECF with buffer ratio of HCO_3^-/CO_2 increased - alkalosis results.

<u>Adverse Effects:</u>

Many of the adverse or toxic effects appear to be secondary to profound effects on electrolyte and water balance.
<u>Excessive loss of potassium</u> – also causes neuromuscular weakness; precipitates arrhythmias and enhances digitalis toxicity.
<u>Hypovolemia</u> – blood volume is decreased sufficiently to decrease blood pressure, reduce renal, cardiac and cerebral blood flow; enhances hypotensive effects of other agents.
<u>Hyperuricemia</u> – increases blood levels of uric acid and may precipitate gouty arthritis.
<u>Hyperglycemia</u> – impaired glucose tolerance.
<u>Ototoxicity</u> – possibly a direct toxic effect on hair cells of cochlea; should not be used with other ototoxic agents (i.e.–aminoglycoside antibiotics, etc.).
<u>Hypersensitivity reactions</u> – blood dyscrasias; azotemia and hepatic encephalopathy may also occur in cirrhotic individuals.

2. <u>Other loop diuretics:</u>

<u>Ethyacrynic Acid</u>

First of the "Loop" diuretics – acts like furosemide, but not a
   sulfonamide derivative.
Get <u>increased excretion of Na^+, Cl^-, K^+ and NH_4^+ and H_2O</u>; diuresis even in
   dehydrated patients with hypovolemia. Can get <u>hypochloremic,
   hypokalemic alkalosis</u>; "contraction alkalosis"

<u>Adverse Effects:</u>
   More GI disturbances than with furosemide but otherwise nearly
   identical to furosemide.

<u>Bumetanide:</u>

   "Loop" diuretic; newer sulfonamide derivative, less frequent otoxicity claimed as its advantage over furosemide.

C. <u>POTASSIUM-SPARING DIURETICS:</u>

1. <u>Aldosterone Antagonist:</u>   <u>Spironolactone is the prototype</u>

   Aldosterone, a steroid secreted by the adrenal cortex, acts on the distal tubule to enhance sodium-potassium exchange mechanism of the renal tubule. Excess aldosterone causes retention of sodium and increased excretion of potassium. The secretion of aldosterone is increased primarily by alterations in electrolyte balance, most importantly by a reduction in effective blood volume, hyponatremia, or hyperkalemia. Secondary hyperaldosteronism is a problem with diuretics – decreased blood volume from diuresis leads to renin release, formation of angiotensin II and consequent stimulation of aldosterone secretion.
   Spironolactone, weak diuretic, usually used in combination with a thiazide or other diuretic – given orally – effects develop slowly (2-3 days); metabolized to an active compound.

<u>Actions</u>:
Competitive antagonism at aldosterone sites in distal tubule and collecting duct; no effect in absence of aldosterone (adrenalectomy). Get <u>increased excretion of sodium</u> and <u>decreased excretion of potassium</u>.

<u>Adverse Effects</u>:
<u>Hyperkalemia</u> - can cause cardiac arrhythmias.
Can cause <u>metabolic acidosis</u> by decreasing secretion of ammonia.
Relatively non-toxic when given alone.
Drowsiness, gynecomastia

2. <u>Other Potassium Sparing Diuretics</u>

<u>Triamterene</u>

Not an aldosterone antagonist, but acts on distal tubule to conserve potassium - action persists after adrenalectomy; orally active - onset of about 1 hour and duration of about 18 hours; partly metabolized, some excreted unchanged. Get <u>sodium diuresis</u> and <u>potassium retention</u>.

<u>Adverse Effects</u>:
<u>Hyperkalemia</u>
Increase in blood urea nitrogen levels
GI disturbances - granulocytopenia
Contraindicated in hepatic and renal insufficiency

<u>Amiloride</u>:

Not an aldosterone antagonist; inhibits electrogenic sodium transport and this affects potassium secretion; decreases K^+ excretion and also decreases Ca^{++} excretion.

<u>Adverse Effects</u>:
Hyperkalemia
GI disturbances
Headache

<u>NOTE</u>: When a potassium sparing diuretic is used potassium supplements are contraindicated.

D. <u>MISCELLANEOUS DRUGS WITH DIURETIC EFFECTS</u>

These drugs have limited therapeutic usefulness and are of historical interest primarily.

<u>Carbonic Anhydrase Inhibitors</u>: <u>Acetazolamide is the prototype</u>.

Organic sulfonamide derivatives; enzyme carbonic anhydrase is specifically inhibited; thought to act primarily at renal proximal tubule to produce the diuretic effect; H_2CO_3 does not break down, Na^+-H^+ exchange does not take place and filtered bicarbonate is excreted instead of being reabsorbed; <u>along with alkaline urine, metabolic acidosis is produced</u> which counteracts diuretic effect.

Clinical usefulness limited primarily to glaucoma. Inhibition of carbonic anhydrase in eye decreases rate of formation of aqueous humor; intraocular pressure decreased.

Osmotic Diuretics: Mannitol is the prototype.

Any inert osmotically active molecule which can be introduced into the blood stream in high concentration, which is freely filtered by the glomeruli, and which is poorly or not reabsorbed by the tubules, will increase urine flow by virtue of the limitation in concentrating ability of the kidney. Not effective in mobilizing edema fluid.

Used to induce water diuresis rather than natriuresis; used in therapy of renal failure to prevent anuria or to maintain a very high urine volume during treatment of intoxication by barbiturates or other agents excreted in urine; also can be used for "dehydrating" action to reduce intracranial pressure or to reduce intraocular pressure.

Xanthines: Theophylline, Aminophylline, Theobromine, and Caffeine

Theophylline is most potent and caffeine the least potent of these agents for a diuretic effect. Increase renal blood flow and glomerular filtration, but also have direct tubular effect and interfere with sodium reabsorption. Diuretic action of xanthine can be a significant side effect. Also have CNS stimulant effects, smooth muscle relaxant effects (bronchodilation and decreased peripheral resistance) and cardiac stimulant effects to increase heart rate and cardiac output; potency differs according to organ system considered.

Mercurial Diuretics: Meralluride, Mercaptomerin, Chlormerodrin

Used rarely. Hg++ (mercuric ion) dissociates in acid environment to react with sulfhydryl groups in enzymes. Inhibits active chloride transport – acts primarily at ascending limb of loop of Henle. Produces hypochloremic alkalosis – alkalosis reduces the renal response to mercury and patients become refractory – ammonium chloride frequently administered to produce acidosis and prevent loss of diuretic effects.

Adverse effects:
Most dangerous effect – induction of cardiac arrhythmias with i.v. use
    (orally – poorly absorbed).
Cytotoxic effects – GI irritation and mucosal necrosis; renal tubular
    necrosis

Dimercaprol (BAL) complexes with mercury to antagonize toxicity of these
    agents.

Acidifying Salts: Ammonium Chloride prototype

Not used for diuresis, but useful for conditions requiring production of acidosis. NH_4Cl converted to urea in liver with release of Cl^-; excess Cl^- retained in plasma at expense of HCO_3^-; results in urinary acidosis.

Uricosuric Diuretics: Attempts to develop a diuretic that would not interfere with urate excretion and cause hyperuricemia are ongoing. No agents currently available in the U.S.

ANTIDIURETIC DRUGS

I. <u>Vasopressin</u> - (See Posterior Pituitary Hormones in Endocrine Section for Additional Information)

    A. Indications:

        1. Treatment of diabetes insipidus of pituitary origin
        2. Treatment of bleeding of esophageal varices
        3. Adjunct in hemophilia therapy - increases circulating levels of blood clotting factor VIII.

    B. Adverse Effects:

        1. Vasoconstriction - may be dangerous in patients with angina
        2. Contraction and cramps of smooth muscles
        3. Water intoxication

    C. Preparations Available:

        1. Desmopressin nasal spray - a synthetic arginine analog with highest ratio of antidiuretic:vasopressor activities and longest duration of action. Drug of choice.
        2. Lypressin nasal spray - a synthetic lysine analog
        3. Vasopressin injection - for i.v. use

II. <u>Other Drugs with Antidiuretic Activity</u>

    A. Clofibrate - An antilipidemic drug, acts by stimulating vasopressin release from the posterior pituitary
    B. Chlorpropamide - An oral hypoglycemic drug, acts by increasing the action of vasopressin on the renal tubule.
    C. Chlorothiazide - Thiazide diuretics paradoxically cause a reduction in polyuria in patients with diabetes insipidus. Chlorothiazide is the drug of choice for nephrogenic diabetes insipidus.

III. <u>Vasopressin Antagonists</u>

    A. Demeclocycline
    B. Lithium carbonate

        1. Both demeclocycline and lithium antagonize the renal action of vasopressin, and are useful in treatment of SIADH (Syndrome of Inappropriate Secretion of Antidiuretic Hormone).

CARDIOVASCULAR DRUGS

CONGESTIVE HEART FAILURE

Digitalis glycosides have been the mainstay of therapy for chronic congestive heart failure (CHF) for centuries. Recently, however, the effectiveness of digitalis glycosides have been questioned in relation to their effect on long term survival benefits. Therapeutic approaches to the treatment of CHF are now being utilized that require a thorough understanding of the pathophysiology of CHF because a) the long term treatment with digitalis of CHF is purely symptomatic, b) significant toxicity occurs in about 10% or more of patients receiving the drug, and c) only about 25% of chronic CHF patients with a normal sinus rhythm are benefited by digitalis.

The primary problem in chronic CHF is decreased ventricular function or contractility; cardiac output is reduced and there is inadequate pumping of blood by the heart to meet the underlying needs of the body. If the underlying cause can be diagnosed and effectively treated by medical or surgical interventions, the failure is reversible. However, when the primary defect is an impairment of the myocardium _per se_, the compensatory mechanisms which affect cardiac output and the ability of the cardiac muscle to function must be considered.

Compensatory mechanisms to improve the low cardiac output may include:

1. Increased preload (EDV - end diastolic volume)
   The Frank-Starling Law of the Heart describes the property of cardiac muscle to increase its contractility as the length of the myocardial fiber (stretch) is increased.
   To accomplish this increase in stretch more blood must be returned to the heart by:
   a. Increased sympathetic tone (discharge) causing vasoconstriction, decreased venous blood storage (pooling), and increased EDV and cardiac output.
   b. Redistribution of blood flow from viscera to heart.
   c. Fluid and Na^+ retention resulting from decreased renal perfusion and renin - angiotensin - aldosterone activation. This increases volume of blood returned to the heart and also may cause edema.
2. Increased heart rate (tachycardia)
   Sympathetic discharge increases rate but this is only helpful within limits as a way of increasing cardiac output.
3. Increased contractility
   Sympathetic discharge increases contractility but only to a limited extent and this may not be enough improvement in contractility to help improve cardiac output in CHF.
4. Decreased impedence (afterload) (blood pressure)
   The marked sympathetic discharge which occurs during compensation increases arteriolar resistance and increases afterload which may speed failure.
5. Cardiac hypertrophy
   Muscle mass increases to improve contractility.

PRELOAD REDUCTION IN CHF

Diuretics - used to decrease edema, reduce blood volume; also may have some action to cause vasodilation. Too vigorous diuresis can be harmful because of excessive reduction of preload and consequent reduction of cardiac output.

<u>Nitrates</u> – produce venous and arterial vasodilation; reduces preload and afterload.

CARDIOTONIC (POSITIVE INOTROPIC) AGENTS

I. <u>DIGITALIS GLYCOSIDES</u>

All useful therapeutic agents are plant steroids; the genin or aglycone is the pharmacologically active principle and consists of the steroid nucleus plus a 5 or 6 membered unsaturated lactone ring at C17 position; saturation of lactone ring reduces the activity; sugars attached at C3 position increase the H_2O solubility, the speed of onset, potency and duration of action; cleavage of lactone ring or removal of –OH at C14 position destroys activity.

<u>Actions:</u>

A. <u>Positive Inotropic Effect</u> – <u>Force of Myocardial Contraction</u>

The fundamental action of digitalis glycosides is to <u>increase the force and velocity</u> of cardiac contractions. The <u>positive inotropic effect is produced</u> both <u>in the normal</u> as well as <u>in the failing heart</u>. When the heart is normal, the increase in myocardial contractility can be demonstrated even though there is no increase in cardiac output. The increased contractility can be detected directly as an <u>increase in the rate of development of tension</u> in the contracting heart (<u>increased dT/dt</u>) or indirectly by demonstrating an <u>increased peak rate of change of the ventricular pressure curve</u> (dP/dt).

It is proposed that digitalis <u>increases contractility by increasing the intracytoplasmic calcium ion concentration</u> during activation by causing an <u>increase in the amount of calcium available for release from the sarcoplasmic reticulum.</u> Thus, more calcium is made available to inhibit the modulatory proteins, troponin and tropomyosin, and thus allow myosin-actin cross bridges to form which permits contraction to proceed. Energy is required for relaxation and myosin-ATPase breaks the cross bridges and allows relaxation to occur as calcium is removed from the modulatory proteins and taken up again by the sarcoplasmic reticulum.

B. <u>Vagal Effects on the Heart</u>

Both <u>direct and vagally mediated slowing of the discharge of the normal pacemaker</u>, the sino-atrial (S-A) node; some slowing of heart rate even in normal individuals if pre-existing vagal tone is not excessive; vagus-dependent component due to stimulation of the vagal nucleus in the medulla or to greater sensitivity of the heart to ACh released on vagal activation (or possibly both factors); <u>vagally mediated component of slowing rate can be abolished by atropine or by vagotomy; the direct component of glycoside action to slow heart rate is not abolished</u> by atropine or by vagotomy. In congestive heart failure, tachycardia occurs as sympathetic activity is increased to compensate; <u>effects of digitalis to slow heart rate are sometimes prominent in congestive heart failure patients when tachycardia exists.</u>

<u>Shortening of the refractory period of atrial muscle</u> – action is apparent only as the speeding of atrial rate during atrial flutter or atrial fibrillation.

<u>Slowing of conduction through the atrio-venticular (A-V) node</u>, causing:
1. Prolonged P-R interval (1° heart block)
2. Dropped beats (2° heart block)
3. Complete atrio-ventricular dissociation (3° heart block)
4. Slowing of ventricular rate during atrial flutter and atrial fibrillation

In patients with atrial fibrillation, ventricular rate depends primarily on the ability of the A-V node to propagate impulses. Since the cardiac glycosides prolong the refractory period of the A-V node, fewer atrial waves of depolarization will reach the ventricles. Consequently ventricular rate will be slowed whether or not the atrial arrhythmias have been altered. The vagal effects of the cardiac glycosides may aid in the termination of atrial arrhythmias <u>per</u> <u>se</u>.

C. <u>Direct Electrophysiological Effects</u>

<u>Atrial muscle</u> – prolongation of refractory period. This direct effect is antagonistic to vagal effect which often dominates to shorten atrial refractory period.

<u>A-V node</u> – slowing of conduction and prolongation of refractory period (direct effect is synergistic with vagal effects to slow conduction and prolong refractory period)

<u>Automaticity</u> – digitalis increases the "automaticity" of secondary latent pacemakers. <u>An abnormal form of automaticity resulting from "afterpotentials" is induced by digitalis. This is the most likely cause of digitalis induced arrthythmias.</u>

Slowing of intracardiac conduction (toxic doses) and increased automaticity lead to:
Extrasystole formation (premature ventricular contractions – particularly likely to occur in diseased hearts)
Production of ventricular tachycardia
Ventricular fibrillation
Asystole (cardiac standstill)

D. <u>Electrocardiographic effects:</u>

Characteristic changes in the ECG produced by digitalis include S-T segment depression, inversion of the T wave, <u>P-R interval prolongation</u> and Q-T interval shortening. Induction or increase of U waves. These sometimes precede signs of toxicity such as bigeminal rhythm, extrasystoles, A-V dissociation and ventricular arrhythmias, etc.

E. <u>Mechanism of Action:</u>

Cardiotonic effect of digitalis is correlated with the ability of glycosides to <u>inhibit the activity of Na^+-K^+ activated ATPase</u>. This effect leads to an <u>increase in intracellular concentrations of Na^+</u>. The elevation in intracellular Na^+ leads to an inhibition of Ca^{2+} extrusion from the cell via a Na^+-Ca^+ exchange pump, resulting in a net increase in intracellular Ca^{2+}. The increase in intracellular Na+ is associated with a corresponding loss in intracellular K^+ and increase in intracellular Ca^{2+}. <u>Toxic effects of glycosides</u> are well correlated to <u>inhibition of the membrane ATPase. Loss of intracellular K^+ favors the induction of arrhythmias</u> during digitalis therapy. <u>However, Ca^{2+} overload induced afterpotentials are the most likely cause of serious arrhythmias.</u>

F. <u>Vascular System</u>:

<u>Direct constrictor effect on arterial and venous smooth muscle.</u> This effect may result in an increase in peripheral resistance and blood pressure (best seen after i.v. administration in normals); despite direct effects of glycosides on vascular smooth muscle, the venous constriction that occurs in congestive heart failure is reversed after treatment with digitalis. The decrease in venous tone and venous pressure follows as a consequence of the improvement of cardiac function and improved hemodynamics and reduction in compensatory sympathetic tone.

G. <u>Gastrointestinal</u>:

Anorexia; nausea; vomiting; diarrhea (central and reflex in nature)

H. <u>Central Nervous System</u>:

Stimulates the vagal nucleus in the medulla – leads to cardiac slowing
   and increase in gastrointestinal motility

Stimulates the chemoreceptor emetic trigger zone in the area postrema
   (floor of the 4th ventricle) – direct chemical stimulation leads to
   nausea and vomiting

Visual changes – changes in color vision; white halos on dark objects

Neurological – headache, <u>fatigue</u>, disorientation, "digitalis delirium"
   seen particularly in the elderly; rare – convulsions; facial pain –
   similar to trigeminal neuralgia

I. <u>Other effects</u>:

Diuresis – primarily the result of increased cardiac function; renal blood flow and increased glomerular filtration result from the improved circulation; digitalis does have secondary effect to inhibit Na^+-K^+ activated ATPase in kidneys as well – not too important in therapy.

<u>Preparations</u>

The major glycosides all have the same therapeutic index

The absorption, distribution and excretion of cardiac glycosides are primarily related to their lipid-water partition coefficient. This, in turn, is determined by the number of hydroxyl groups attached to the genin.

<u>Digoxin</u>: (two genin hydroxyls) less lipid soluble, more water soluble than digitoxin
>   half-life = 36 hrs (dependent on renal function)
>   60-85% absorbed from G.I. tract
>   25% bound to plasma protein
>   Excreted primarily unchanged in the urine
>   Onset (i.v. loading) = 15-30 min
>   Peak = 1-5 hrs.

<u>Digitoxin</u>: Most lipid soluble with only one genin hydroxyl group.

>   half-life = 5-7 days (not dependent on renal function)
>   90-100% absorbed from the G.I. tract
>   97% bound to plasma protein
>   Metabolized almost completely in the liver
>   Onset (with i.v. loading dose) = 1/2 - 2 hrs
>   Peak = 4-12 hrs.
>   Therapeutic plasma levels = 14-26 ng/ml

<u>Other Preparations</u>

<u>Lanatoside C</u> - duration similar to digoxin, but poor oral absorption
<u>Ouabain</u> - short acting, only used experimentally
<u>Acetylstrophanthidin</u> - ultra-short acting, only used experimentally
<u>Digitalis leaf</u> (whole leaf preparation) - duration similar to digitoxin, but 1/1000 as potent

<u>Administration</u>

Each patient should be "titrated" to achieve a balance between elimination of the drug and cumulative effects; try to achieve adequate therapeutic effects and minimize undesirable side effects or outright toxicity.

<u>Digitalizing dose vs. maintenance dose</u>: Traditionally, digitalis administered in large doses (priming doses) to achieve high plasma concentration and tissue saturation - followed by smaller doses to maintain plasma levels. Only in an <u>emergency</u> situation is this now thought to be necessary. Now a slower method of administration is recommended - the smaller maintenance dose can be given over several half-lives until the desired serum digitalis level is achieved. This method allows digitalization to occur with less likelihood of toxicity - the patient can be observed frequently as the digitalization is proceeding. With digoxin, $t_{\frac{1}{2}}$ of 1.5 days, a steady state serum digitalis level would be achieved in about 7 days. Four to five half-lives are sufficient to produce a steady state in which the amount metabolized and excreted balances that absorbed.

<u>Desirable effects to be achieved with digitalis therapy</u>
In congestive heart failure - increase cardiac output; reduction of circulating blood volume and elimination of edema fluid; venous pressure

is reduced; cardiac size is decreased; the heart rate decreases (if increase was due to CHF).

In atrial fibrillation – reduction of the ventricular rate to below 80.

<u>Toxic Effects of Digitalis</u>

Differences between the therapeutic and toxic levels is very small, especially if maximal contractile effects are sought. All preparations have the same therapeutic index.

The major common cause of toxicity is cellular Ca^{2+} overload.
Toxicity is exacerbated by: Sympathomimetic agents, $\uparrow Ca^{++}$, $\downarrow Mg^{++}$, hypoxia, increased heart rate, and most commonly K^+ depletion. Beware of the varied clinical situations which may cause the above conditions.

<u>Anorexia</u>, <u>fatigue</u>, headache, nausea, neuralgic pain and altered color vision (yellow hues) are some side effects which may occur prior to, simultaneously with or after more serious arrhythmias due to cardiac glycoside toxicity.

<u>Treatment of Toxicity</u>

1. Discontinue cardiac glycosides
2. Correct precipitating factors (eg., electrolyte disturbances)
3. Treat serious arrhythmias
    -potassium salts with normal renal function and constant monitoring
    -antiarrhythmic drugs with care
    -asystole may result in presence of complete heart block and abolition of ventricular arrhythmia
4. Steroid binding resins (primarily for digitoxin) and digoxin specific antibodies may be useful to aid drug removal.

<u>Precautions:</u>

Cardioversion should be used only as a last resort if digitalis toxicity is suspected. Cardioversion (DC countershock) precipitates digitalis-induced arrhythmias. Digitalis should be discontinued in advance of cardioversion.

Glycosides and calcium act synergistically – calcium salts can precipitate arrhythmias in digitalized patient; EDTA (chelating agent) has been used to chelate Ca^{++} and to lower serum Ca^{++} levels in digitalis arrhythmias – not useful clinically.

Several drugs including quinidine have been shown to increase cardiac glycoside serum levels. Concurrent use of these agents require caution to avoid toxicity.

<u>Uses:</u>

Digitalis is often used prior to quinidine administration in atrial flutter or fibrillation. Used to protect the ventricles from rapid atrial discharges by prolonging the refractory period of the AV node and slowing conduction of impulses through the AV node.

     <u>Congestive Heart Failure</u>: digitalis by enhancing the force of contraction of the ventricle, significantly increases cardiac output, decreases right atrial pressure and increases the excretion of Na^+ and H_2O; decreases circulating blood volume. Heart rate (frequently very fast during failure) is reduced; venous pooling is increased and venous return to the heart is decreased.

II.   <u>BETA-ADRENERGIC RECEPTOR AGONISTS</u>: Dopamine, dobutamine and isoproterenol.

     Role of these agents in treatment of chronic CHF remains to be demonstrated.

     The positive inotropic effects of these <u>beta</u>-agonists have been proven useful for the treatment of acute CHF; given parenterally to increase cardiac contractility; vasodilator effects may also be useful.

III. <u>AMRINONE</u>:

     Positive inotropic agent with vasodilator activity; mechanism of action is unknown. Used parenterally for the short term management of CHF in patients who have not responded to digitalis, preload or afterload reduction.

     Hepatotoxicity, reversible thrombocytopenia, GI disturbances and hypersensitivity reactions have been reported.

<u>AFTERLOAD REDUCTION</u>

    <u>Vasodilators</u>: reduction in peripheral resistance can increase stroke volume.

      <u>Hydralazine</u>: a direct vasodilator (See antihypertensive section) effectivenss is questionable

      <u>Prazosin</u>: an $alpha_1$ receptor antagonist (See antihypertensive section) effectiveness is questionable

      <u>Captopril</u>: angiotensin-converting enzyme inhibitor; approved for use in CHF for its afterload reducing effect, but side effects may limit its usefulness (See autacoids section).

ANTIARRHYTMIC DRUGS

Cardiac arrhythmias result from abnormal impulse formation (automaticity), abnormal impulse conduction or some combination of these two mechanisms.

Abnormal automaticity

1. S.A. node discharges too fast or too slow
2. Accessory pacemakers may be faster than abnormally slow SA node or be abnormally fast and usurp control of the cardiac rhythm.
3. Abnormal pacemakers may be induced by injury or stretch.

Abnormal conduction

1. Reentry arrhythmias – impulse traverses circuitous path and reexcites the myocardium repetitively. Unidirectional block of the impulse and slow conduction/short refractory period are required for this model.
2. Impulse is blocked or slowed along normal conduction path leading to delayed activation of some areas of the myocardium.

Antiarrhythmic drugs have been grouped based on general concepts of their major mechanisms of action. These groupings have changed over the years. The more current grouping is given below.

Group IA: quinidine, procainamide, disopyramide

These agents decrease automaticity, depress conduction velocity and excitability of the normal and abnormal myocardium and increase the action potential duration (APD) and effective refractory period (ERP).

Group IB: lidocaine, phenytoin

Historically believed to increase cardiac conduction velocity, these agents are now thought to selectively depress or abolish conduction in injured, slightly depolarized excitable tissues. Normal tissue is not depressed at therapeutic concentrations. APD and ERP are decreased and automaticity is depressed.

Group IC: flecainide, encainide

Depression of conduction velocity with no change in APD or ERP.

Group II: propranolol, β-blocking agents

These agents are β-receptor blocking drugs which depress conduction and contractility. They decrease APD, ERP and automaticity.

Group III: Bretyllium, sotalol amiodarone

The major characteristic of this group is marked prolongation of APD and ERP.

Group IV: Verapamil and other Ca^{++} antagonists.

This group of agents is comprised of blockers of the slow inward (Ca^{++} mediated, I_{si}) current. They are thought to act by completely blocking conduction in partially depolarized tissues which are excitable only due to I_{si} or in nodal tissue. These agents are most effective in atrial or nodal arrhythmias.

<u>New antiarrhythmic agents</u>

Many newer agents are now available or may become clinically important in a few years because of some unique properties. These include:

a) Orally effective, lidocaine-like: mexilitine, tocainide
b) Quinidine-like: aprindine, ethmozin
c) Action potential prolonging agents: amiodarone, sotalol

QUINIDINE (Group IA)

The d-isomer of quinine; well absorbed orally; dangerous hypotensive agent i.v., hydroxylated by the liver; up to 50% excreted as unchanged drug.

<u>Cardiac Actions:</u>

Depresses intracardiac conduction (reduces responsiveness of cardiac cell
    membrane to stimulation and hence decreases conduction velocity - slow
    depolarization rate of phase 0 of action potential and decreases amplitude
    of action potential), ↑ QRS duration (marked prolongation requires
    withdrawal of drug or asystole may ensue)
Decreases automaticity (decreases rate of slow diastolic, phase 4
    depolarization) more depression of ectopic, premature beats than of
    normally spaced beats
Directly-prolongs action potential and refractory periods of cardiac tissues
Depresses myocardial contractility (important if the myocardium is already
    weak)
Weak cholinergic blocking action (atropine-like effect) - can cause a
    paradoxical increase in ventricular rate by speeding rate of discharge of
    SA node (by blocking vagal-induced tone) and by increasing conduction
    velocity through the AV node (also by blocking vagal-induced slowing of
    conduction through node)

Other effects:
    Relaxation of vascular smooth muscle - hypotension
    Nausea, vomiting, diarrhea - a frequent problem
    Cinchonism (salivation, tinnitus, vertigo, headache, visual disturbances,
        confusion) - seen with chronic use and toxicity
    Thrombocytopenic purpura - rare but serious
    Can cause ↑ in serum cardiac glycoside levels and increase glycoside
        toxicity.
    May cause paradoxical ventricular tachycardia in atrial flutter
    May cause ventricular fibrillation
    May cause asystole

Often used for the treatment of: Atrial premature contractions
                                  Prophylactic management of atrial fibrillation
                                      (but digitalize first to avoid the
                                      possibility of increasing the ventricular
                                      rate due to a slowing of atrial automaticity
                                      (direct effect) while AV conduction is
                                      enhanced (atropine-like effect)

PROCAINAMIDE (Group IA)

Amide derivative of local anesthetic, procaine; amide link prevents rapid hydrolysis by plasma esterases; can be given orally or i.v.; procainamide is more suitable than quinidine for i.v. administration; 60% excreted unchanged; renal insufficiency – dangerous.

<u>Cardiac Actions</u>: Like quinidine; decreases automaticity, decreases membrane responsiveness; prolongs refractory period; depresses intracardiac conduction; also has weak atropine-like cholinergic blocking action; decreases myocardial contractility.

Other effects:
Relaxes vascular smooth muscle – hypotension
Causes a syndrome which resembles systemic lupus erythematosis (SLE)
Can cause agranulocytosis; skin rashes
Nausea, vomiting, confusion, hallucinations, chills and fever reported

DISOPYRAMIDE (Group IA)

Very similar to quinidine but better tolerated orally. Marked anticholinergic effects. Depresses myocardial contractilty. Other effects similar to quinidine <u>without</u> cinchonism.

LIDOCAINE (Group IB)

A local anesthetic; only given i.v. – infusion permits moment-to-moment control; primarily metabolized by liver; use cautiously in hepatic disease.

<u>Cardiac Actions</u>: Classically thought to increase membrane responsiveness – may enhance intracardiac conduction in some circumstances if it is previously depressed with low potassium permeability (in this special circumstance it increases depolarization rate of phase 0 of the action potential and increases amplitude of the action potential).
Decreases automaticity (decreases phase 4 depolarization) – suppresses
    extrasystole formation.
Selectively depresses or blocks conduction in injured or slightly depolarized
    myocardium. Shortens APD and ERP.
Generally useful for ventricular arrthythmias only.
Other effects:
Cardiac depression at high doses or following other antiarrhythmic agents.
Hypotension
Drowsiness, paresthesias, decreased auditory acuity, disorientation
Respiratory depression, twitching, agitation, convulsions

PHENYTOIN (Group IB)

Anticonvulsant absorbed after oral administration; also given i.v.; almost completely metabolized – metabolites excreted.

<u>Cardiac Actions</u>: Actions similar to lidocaine, but longer acting.

Other Effects:
    CV – hypotension, cardiac depression at high concentrations or following
        other antiarrhythmic agents

CNS – nystagmus, ataxia, vertigo, drowsiness, nausea
Megaloblastic anemia and lymphoma-like syndrome

FLECAINIDE AND ENCAINIDE (Group IC)

These agents depress conduction in normal and abnormal cardiac tissue like
group IA agents. However, they do not exert much effect on APD or ERP. None are
currently approved for use in the United States.

PROPRANOLOL (Group II)

Has two different antiarrhythmic actions (β blocking effect deemed most
important):

> <u>Beta</u> adrenergic blocking effect, useful in opposing the actions of
> catecholamines released by the sympatho-adrenal system;
> pheochromocytoma; epinephrine-anesthetic induced arrhythmias.
> Primarily useful for atrial arrhythmias
> <u>Direct effect</u> upon myocardial cell membrane (at doses greater than those
> required for <u>beta</u>-adrenergic blocking effect; decreases automaticity,
> decreases membrane responsiveness; depresses intracardiac conduction –
> but also shortens APD and ERP like group IB agents.

Other Effects:
Cardiac depression – can precipitate congestive heart failure
Depresses AV nodal conduction
Can cause hypotension
Can cause asystole (depression of AV conduction plus suppression of
ventricular automaticity
Bronchoconstriction or spasm
Other blocking agents are similar (except Sotalol-see below)

BRETYLLIUM (Group III)

Primarily known for prolonging APD and ERP but also has an antiadrenergic
mechanism; used only in hospital for refractory ventricular arrhythmias

Other Effects:
Hypotension, hypersensitivity to vasopressors

SOTALOL (Group III)

This β blocking drug markedly prolongs APD and ERP of the cardiac conducting
system (thus classification as a group III agent).

AMIODARONE (Group III)

Newly approved agent which markedly prolongs APD and ERP. This effect occurs
slowly over a period of weeks. Depresses conduction velocity and is a
vasodilator. Acutely prolongs A.V. nodal refractory period and slows A.V.
conduction with I.V. administration.
This agent has a wide variety of side effects with prolonged administration
and its use is limited to life threatening, refractory arrhythmias for this
reason. Toxic effects include pulmonary toxicity, liver toxicity, corneal

microdeposits, photosensitivity, altered thyroid function, life threatening arrhythmias.

VERAPAMIL (Group IV)

Calcium channel blocking agent useful for supraventricular arrhythmias. Major problems include predisposition to heart failure and depression of A.V. nodal conduction. See calcium antagonist section for further details.

General considerations for bradyarrhythmias

In severe bradycardia, there is danger of extrasystole formation and fibrillation. Furthermore, the bradycardia may limit cardiac output. Therefore, there may be occasions to employ:
    Atropine: To block cardiac muscarinic receptors to prevent excess vagal
        slowing
    Isoproterenol: To stimulate beta adrenergic receptors of the cardiac
        pacemaker cells.

NOTE: Electrical devices now do some of the jobs which were formerly attempted with drugs.
    Cardioversion - for most tachyarrhythmias
    Pacemakers   - for bradycardia and heart block

ANTI-ANGINAL DRUGS

Drugs used in the treatment of angina pectoris: synonyms – anti-anginal, coronary "vasodilators".

<u>Angina pectoris</u> – a chronic disease characterized by intermittent attacks of chest pain, associated with exertion, stress, excitement and other factors which can increase cardiac work.

Although the pathophysiology of angina pectoris has defied precise definition, it is generally accepted that the syndrome of angina pectoris results from myocardial ischemia, whether due to coronary artery disease, tachycardia, aortic valvular disease, thyrotoxicosis, anemia, coronary arteriovenous fistula or impaired hemoglobin-O_2 dissociation.

<u>Varient or Prinzmetal's angina</u> – often occurs at rest due to coronary arterial spasm.

<u>Pain</u> – result of relative ischemia of areas of myocardium in which the metabolic demand for O_2 (due to increased cardiac work) has outstripped the capacity of the coronary circulation to provide arterial (oxygenated) blood.

Evaluation of all treatment programs, medical or surgical, is most difficult because the pain is influenced by so many factors, particularly emotional ones. However, it is agreed that the design of satisfactory therapy for angina must include:
1. Reduction of the frequency and severity of attacks of chest pain
2. Removal of any underlying cause, if possible
3. Promotion of growth of collateral vessels
4. Prevention of sudden death

<u>Ideal Goal of Therapy</u>: To dilate narrowed coronary vessels and permit more adequate perfusion of working myocardium. Unfortunately, it appears that in cases of conventional angina, (angina on exertion) coronary narrowing is structural (atheromatous – "lead pipe" vessels) and can not be corrected by vasodilation. Therefore, a second therapeutic goal may be more realistic – reduction of cardiac work to within the limits appropriate for the available coronary flow. Vasodilators or antispasmotics are required for therapy of Prinzmetal's angina.

Cardiac work and myocardial O_2 demand can be decreased by:

a) decreased preload
b) decreased afterload
c) decreased contractility
d) decreased rate
e) decreased sympathetic tone which influences all of the above

A. <u>Nitrates and nitrites</u> – smooth muscle relaxants (vasodilators)

Although nitrates cause general vasodilatation, relief of anginal pain is not believed to be related to coronary artery dilatation and increased coronary blood flow, but rather to the effectiveness of nitrates in reducing cardiac workload. The drugs reduce systemic and pulmonary arterial and venus pressures and decrease cardiac output. Nitrates should be used judiciously in glaucoma and in conditions with increased intracranial pressure. They should be used cautiously in patients with acute myocardial infarction because of their tendency to produce hypotension.

The only other important effect of this group is the conversion of hemoglobin to methemoglobin by excessively high serum nitrite levels. Since nitrates can be reduced in the gut to nitrites, nitrate drugs also can cause methemoglobinemia. This effect is used to treat cyanide intoxication.

Tolerance to the cardiovascular effects of these agents is a problem with continuous prophylaxis.

<u>Rapidly acting preparations for acute attacks:</u>

1. <u>Glyceryl trinitrate (nitroglycerin)</u>: prototype

    Dispensed in tablets; should be dissolved sublingually; act within 2-3 min; duration of action about 20 minutes.

    <u>Unpleasant side effects:</u>

    Includes sensations of warmth, flushing, throbbing headaches, and varying degrees of dizziness, postural hypotension and syncope. Occassionally with the first dose, nitroglycerin may produce enough postural hypotension to result in paradoxical angina (hypotension may cause reflex tachycardia and increased contractility which increases workload and brings on anginal attack). In these cases, patients should lie down when taking the nitrate.

2. <u>Amyl nitrite</u>: volatile liquid, available in glass "pearls" or ampules; administered by inhalation; onset about 10 seconds; duration about 5-10 minutes.

<u>Long acting preparations for prophylaxis:</u>

The clinical effectiveness of such oral or topical preparations is disputed; the onset of their effects after single doses is delayed for 15 – 60 minutes, but persists for several hours; repeated doses may lead to tolerance and the results of clinical trials are at best conflicting. The placebo effect to decrease anxiety of expected attacks may be beneficial however.

Pentaerythrityl tetranitrate
Erythrityl tetranitrate
Isosorbide dinitrate

C. <u>Propranolol</u>

A <u>beta</u>-adrenergic blocking agent that is becoming one of the drugs of choice for prophylaxis against conventional angina on exertion. It decreases heart rate, cardiac output, mean aterial pressure, left ventricular work and O_2 consumption. Although it has been found to decrease the episodes of pain in angina, it generally does not normalize ischemic ST segment depression. Can precipitate congestive heart failure; bronchoconstriction; can aggravate angina in some patients. Not generally effective for Prinzmetal's angina.

More selective <u>beta</u>$_1$ receptor antagonists appear to have less extracardiac side effects.

D. <u>Calcium antagonists</u>

<u>Nifedipine</u>
<u>Diltiazem</u>
     Currently approved agents for prophylaxis of angina pectoris.
Vasodilators and may decrease contractility somewhat. These actions are caused by
a direct antagonism of Ca^{++} entry into the cell. Major drawback - may predispose
to heart failure by decreasing contractility.

E. <u>Dipyridamole</u>

     Coronary vasodilator which appears effective in varient agina due to
vasospasm, but not conventional angina due to atherosclerosis.

* * * * * * * * * *

<u>Treatment of cyanide poisoning</u>

     Amyl nitrite or sodium nitrite, the principal agents which cause the formation
of methemoglobin, are used in the treatment of cyanide intoxication.

     Cyanide, which poisons tissue cytochromes, also has an affinity for
methemoglobin and forms cyanmethemoglobin; the formation of cyanmethemoglobin
liberates the cytochromes and allows tissue respiration to proceed.

     The cyanide which is subsequently slowly released from cyanmethemoglobin may
then be converted to a thiocyanate by the coadministration of thiosulfate with the
nitrite.

CALCIUM CHANNEL BLOCKERS

Calcium channel blockers (calcium antagonists, calcium entry or slow channel blockers) all inhibit or block the movement (influx) of calcium ions across the cell membrane through voltage-activated slow channels (I_{si}). The cardiovascular consequences of this action are summarized in the table.

These agents differ in their spectrum and selectivity of effects on the heart and blood vessels. For example, although these agents will have a hypotensive effect, the magnitude of the vasodilator effect differs and this determines the magnitude of the reflex sympathetic response to counteract the hypotension.

Calcium channel blockers dilate coronary arteries and are useful in inhibiting the coronary artery spasm of variant or Prinzmetal's angina, thereby improving blood flow to the myocardium. The vasodilating effect on systemic arteries and the reduction of peripheral vascular resistance reduces the workload of the heart which decreases the oxygen and energy requirements. The direct negative inotropic effects of the calcium channel blockers also contribute to the decreased myocardial oxygen requirements.

	Nifedipine	Verapamil	Diltiazem
Cardiac Electrophysiology			
AV node conduction velocity	0/–[1]	---	--
Ventricular conduction velocity	0	0	0
AV node ERP	0/+[1]	++	+
Ventricular ERP	0	0	0
SA node automaticity	0/–[1]	--	–
Ventricular automaticity	0	0	0
Antiarrhythmic activity	0	+++	0
Hemodynamics			
Myocardial contractility	0/–[1]	--	–
Peripheral resistance (afterload)	---	--	–
Venous capcitance (preload)	0	0	0
Antianginal activity	++	++	++[2]
Antihypertensive	++	+	0/+

1. Net effect depends on autonomic reflexes to peripheral vasodilation.
2. Vasospastic angina (Prinzmetal's) more than classic angina.

Verapamil: Well absorbed; significant first-pass metabolism; constipation; headache; contraindicated in CHF patients or those with AV conduction disturbances because of its negative inotropic effect.

Nifedipine: Well absorbed; the most effective vasodilator; the common side effects (headache, hypotension, reflex tachycardia, flushing, pedal edema) are related to vasodilator action.

Diltiazem: Well absorbed; headache, nausea and pedal edema reported; liver enzymes elevated in some patients.

DRUGS USED IN THE TREATMENT OF HYPERLIPOPROTEINEMIAS

I. Clofibrate

    A. Lowers VLDL and plasma triglycerides.
    B. Mechanism unclear (cholesterol synthesis in liver is inhibited but this does not explain triglyceride-lowering effect).
    C. Drug of choice for type III hyperlipidemia; may also be used for types IIb, IV and V.
    D. Contraindicated in patients with impaired renal or hepatic function.
    E. Adverse effects: GI disturbances, muscle weakness.
    F. Displaces acidic drugs from plasma proteins; reduction in the dose of anticoagulant is required.
    G. May increase LDL levels; an indication to stop its use.
    H. Long term-increased incidence of thromboembolism, angina, arrhythmias, gallstones. No evidence of benefit in CAHD.

II. Cholestyramine + Colestipol

    A. Lower LDL and plasma cholesterol.
    B. Bind bile acids in gut; increased hepatic conversion of cholesterol to bile acids.
    C. Steroid binding resins; not absorbed.
    D. Adverse effects: Unpleasant taste and smell, constipation, steatorrhea, deficiency of fat-soluble vitamins (e.g., K).
    E. May adsorb other drugs given concurrently.
    F. Drug of choice for type IIa hyperlipidemia; with niacin for type IIb.

III. Nicotinic Acid (Niacin)

    A. Lowers both cholesterol and triglycerides.
    B. Mechanisms: inhibits triglyceride lipase activation by lipolytic hormones; reduces LDL synthesis.
    C. Adverse effects: flushing, GI irritation, activation of peptic ulcer, abnormal hepatic function, hyperglycemia, hyperuricemia.
    D. Limited to high-risk patients not responding to other drugs (Types II, III, IV, V)

IV. Gemfibrozil

    A. Lowers serum triglycerides; sometimes increases HDL
    B. Mechanism is decreased VLDL synthesis
    C. Similar to clofibrate in most respects

V. Probucol

    A. Decreases LDL and cholesterol
    B. Inhibits cholesterol synthesis
    C. Side effects include diarrhea, flatence, nausea, abdominal pain
    D. Long persistance in adipose tissue

VI. Others - Rarely used

ANTIHYPERTENSIVE THERAPY

1. Clearly reduces cerebrovascular disease, heart failure, renal insufficiency and possibly the risk of myocardial infarction.
2. Is indicated whenever:
   a) target organs are affected;
   b) minimally elevated blood pressure is associated with other cardiovascular risk factors; e.g., smoking, diabetes, obesity, hyperlipidemia and genetic predisposition;
   c) persistent blood pressure elevations above 145/90 or 170-180/95 in the elderly.
3. May initially consist of reducing salt intake and weight, and modification of other risk factors.
4. "Step Therapy" is appropriate in many patients.
   Step I - usually a thiazide diuretic. (May also be beta blocker or converting enzyme inhibitor in certain patients). If inadequate add:
   Step II - an antiadrenergic (methyldopa, clonidine, prazosin, reserpine) or a beta-adrenergic blocker. If this is inadequate add:
   Step III - a vasodilator (hydralazine, prazosin or minoxidil).

Mechanism of Action		Drug Category	Drugs
Diuretics	a)	Thiazides and related agents	Chlorothiazide (Diuril) Chlorthalidone (Hygroton)
	b)	Loop diuretics	Furosemide (Lasix) Ethacrynic acid (Edocrin) Bumethanide (Bumex)
	c)	Potassium-sparing diuretics	Triamterine (Dyrenium) Spironolactone (Aldactone) Amiloride (Midamor)
Sympatolytic Drugs	a)	Centrally acting agents	Clonidine (Catapres) Methyldopa (Aldomet) Guanabenz (Wytensen)
	b)	Beta-adrenergic antagonists	Propranolol (Inderal) Metaprolol (Lopressor) Nadolol (Corgard) Atenolol (Tenormin) Pindolol (Visken) Timolol (Blocadren)
	c)	Alpha-adrenergic antagonists	Prazosin (Minipress) Phenoxybenzamine (Dibenzyline) Phentolamine (Regitine)
	d)	Mixed antagonists	Labetalol (Normodyne, Trandate, Vescal)
	e)	Adrenergic neuron blocking agents	Reserpine (Serpasil) Guanethidine (Ismelin)
	f)	MAO-inhibitor	Pargyline (Eutonyl)
	g)	Ganglionic blocking agents	Trimethaphan (Arfonad) Mecamylamine (Inversin)
Direct Vasodilators	a)	Arterial vasodilators	Hydralazine (Apresoline) Minoxidil (Loniten) Diazoxide (Hyperstat)
	b)	Calcium antagonists	Diltiazem (Cardizem) Nifedipine (Procardia) Verapamil (Isoptin, Calan)
	c)	Arterial and venous vasodilator	Sodium nitropusside (Nipride, Nitropress)
Angiotensin Antagonists	a)	Converting enzyme inhibitors	Captropril (Capoten) Enalapril (Vasotec)
	b)	Angiotensin II receptor blocker	Saralasin (Sarenin)

A. <u>Baroreceptor Reflex Inhibitors of Sympathetic Function</u>

    1. <u>Veratrum alkaloids</u>:
        a. Sensitize baroreceptors and activate the afferent nerve endings
            causing reflex mechanisms to lower blood pressure and heart rate (and
            in larger doses, also produces apnea); activates the Bezold-Jarisch
            reflex (vagal-vagal)
        b. Not used now because of side effects; also produces tolerance and
            emesis.

B. <u>Hypotensive Diuretics</u>

    1. <u>Sulfonamide Diuretics (Thiazides, Chlorothiazide, Hydrochlorothiazide)</u>:
        a. Orally effective - useful for mild to moderate hypertension; standard
            now in therapy of hypertension; frequently given along with other
            antihypertensive medication and can potentiate the action of other
            antihypertensive drugs.
        b. Precise mode of action poorly understood; antihypertensive effects
            during the first few weeks of treatment have been related to decreased
            circulating blood volume and decreased cardiac output, but these
            return to nearly normal values after a few weeks; action may in part
            be related to a depletion or redistribution of sodium; may act by
            direct arteriolar dilation.
        c. Antihypertensive actions of all thiazides are comparable.
        d. K^+ loss leads to hypokalemic alkalosis; rarely a problem in normal
            patients; may be problematic in patients with cardiac arrhythmias,
            especially if on digitalis or those with severe liver disease.
        e. Some increase in plasma lipid concentrations.

    2. <u>Loop Diuretics (Furosemide, Ethacrynic Acid, Bumethanide)</u>:
        a. More potent with more potential for side effects; increased renin;
            hypokalemia; hyperglycemia; hyperuricemia
        b. Thiazides more effective than loop diuretics in patients without
            edema.

    3. <u>Potassium-Sparing Diuretics</u>:
        a. <u>Spironolactone</u>: As effective as thiazides but more side effects. May
            be useful in patients with hyperuricemia, hypokalemia, glucose
            intolerance. Drug of choice in patients with primary aldosteronism.
        b. <u>Triamterene and Amiloride</u>: May be given along with the thiazide to
            prevent potassium depletion (have little hypotensive action alone).

C. <u>Sympatholytic Drugs</u>

    1. <u>CNS Sympatho-Inhibitory Drugs</u>:

        a. <u>Clonidine</u>:
            1. CNS stimulation of <u>alpha$_2$</u>-adrenoceptors causes inhibition of
                sympathetic tone. Effects antagonized by yohimbine; long acting.
            2. Very lipophylic; orally administered; may be given with
                transdermal patch.
            3. Side effects include xerostomia (dry mouth); sedation; fluid
                retention (use with diuretic).
            4. Withdrawal may precipitate hypertensive crisis; may be treated
                with labetalol, <u>beta</u> antagonist.

b. <u>Methyldopa</u>:
   1. Metabolized to <u>alpha</u>-methyl norepinephrine (<u>alpha</u>-MNE) which can
      displace and deplete NE in storage sites; research indicates that
      the antihypertensive effect is central; causes drowsiness and
      depression; may act on CNS <u>alpha</u>-2 receptors to decrease
      sympathetic tone by <u>alpha</u>-MNE (indirect decrease of renin
      release).

c. <u>Guanabenz</u>: Like clonidine.

2. <u>Beta-Adrenergic Receptor Blocking Agents</u> (see details in section II):

   a. <u>Propranolol</u>:
      1) Non-selective <u>beta</u>$_1$ and <u>beta</u>$_2$ blocker.
      2) Mechanism of action: decreases cardiac output; decreases
         sympathetic tone <u>via</u> central action and decrease renin release.
      3) Adverse effects: bradycardia, congestive heart failure, mental
         depression and bronchospasm.

   b. <u>Nadolol</u>:
      1) Non-selective <u>beta</u>$_1$ and <u>beta</u>$_2$ blocker but lacks direct myocardial
         depressant effect as propranolol.
      2) Long duration of action; can be used once a day,
      3) Mechanism of action: similar to propranolol.
      4) Adverse effects: bradycardia, dizziness, bronchospasm and cardiac
         failure.

   c. <u>Metoprolol and Atenolol</u>:
      1) More selective <u>beta</u>$_1$ blocker (cardiac selective).
      2) Mechanism of action: similar to propranolol.
      3) Adverse effects: headache, insomnia, dizziness.
      4) Precaution: could be used in asthmatics for treatment of
         hypertension but requires caution.

   d. <u>Pindolol</u>:
      1) Non-selective
      2) Indirect sympathomimetic activity (ISA); less cardiac depression
         at rest
      3) Adverse effects as above

   e. <u>Timolol</u>:
      1) Nonselective
      2) Drug of choice in open angle glaucoma
      3) Adverse effects as above

3. <u>Alpha-adrenergic receptor blocking agents</u>: (See details in section II)
   a. Trials with phenoxybenzamine and phentolamine have been generally
      disappointing.
   b. Adverse effects, such as orthostatic hypotension, tachycardia, etc.,
      make these drugs clinically unacceptable for treating hypertension.
   c. <u>Exception</u>: May be useful during surgical removal of pheochromocytoma
      to prevent excessive hypertension caused by the release of
      catecholamines during surgical manipulation of the tumor.
   d. <u>Prazosin</u>: A newly released antihypertensive drug which acts
      selectively on the post-synaptic <u>alpha</u>$_1$ receptor of vascular smooth

muscle. Orthostatic hypotension and reflex tachycardia are not as prominent as with other <u>alpha</u>-blockers.

4. <u>Mixed Antagonist</u>:
   a. <u>Labetalol</u>: (See details in section II).

5. <u>Adrenergic Neuron Blockers</u>:
   a. <u>Reserpine</u>:
      1. Depletes NE stores by preventing uptake and storage in neurosecretory granules - appears to act by inhibiting transport and binding of catecholamines in storage granules; depletes both in peripheral sympathetics and in the brain.
      2. Get unopposed parasympathetic effects - bradycardia, nasal stuffiness, GI effects (diarrhea, increased motility, aggravation of peptic ulcers).
      3. Other adverse effects: excessive sedation, depression, extrapyramidal symptoms, impotence.

   b. <u>Guanethidine</u>:
      1. Complex actions on the adrenergic neuron; prevents NE release when nerve is stimulated by blocking transmission of the action potential into the terminal nerve ending; also can deplete peripheral stores of NE and block reuptake of NE; does not cross blood-brain-barrier; no CNS effect.
      2. Slow onset (2-3 days) with long duration of action (effects persist for about a week after drug is stopped).
      3. Causes postural hypotension, bradycardia, diarrhea, nasal stuffiness, failure of ejaculation.

6. <u>Monoamine oxidase (MAO) inhibitors</u>
   a. <u>Pargyline</u>: synthesized for use in hypertension. Through complex feedback mechanism, allows the build up of a false transmitter, octopamine, in nerve endings; may produce serious side effects - marked postural hypotension, danger of producing hypertensive crisis (interaction with tyramine containing foods, other drugs).

7. <u>Ganglionic Blocking Agents</u>
   a. Very potent antihypertensive drugs; block transmission of impulses through ganglia of the autonomic nervous system; interfere with the action of ACh on the ganglion cells; produces parasympathetic as well as sympathetic block.
   b. Hypotensive action is primarily due to reduced vasomotor tone, decreased venous return and lowered cardiac output
   c. Now rarely used because of side effects
   d. <u>Trimethaphan</u>: Occasionally used for hypertensive crisis; given by slow i.v. drip; dangerous drug - can cause precipitous fall in blood pressure; also causes histamine release.

D. <u>Direct Vasodilators</u>

   1. <u>Hydralazine</u>:
      a. Direct relaxant of vascular smooth muscle to decrease peripheral resistance.
      b. Reflex cardiac stimulation (increased cardiac output and tachycardia) can be blocked by administration of propranolol.
      c. Well absorbed after oral administration and generally well tolerated for treatment of chronic hypertension; useful in acute hypertensive crisis (parenteral).
      d. Adverse effects: Headache, palpitations, GI disturbances; most serious toxicity is a lupus-like syndrome occurring with long term therapy; this is reversible if drug stopped: this side effect limits its chronic use.

   2. <u>Minoxidil</u>:
      a. Long acting direct dilator of vascular smooth muscle.
      b. Reflex cardiac stimulation.
      c. Adverse effects: salt and water retention and hypertrichosis (growth of hair).
      d. Reserved for more severe and uncontrollable hypertension.

   3. <u>Diazoxide</u>:
      a. A non-diuretic congener of the thiazide diuretic drugs.
      b. Precise mechanism of action unknown, but exerts direct effect on the arterioles to lower blood pressure.
      c. Given i.v. for acute hypertensive emergencies.
      d. Adverse effects: Hyperglycemia (inhibits insulin release from the <u>beta</u> cells of the pancreas), hyperuricemia, amylase elevations and even pancreatic necrosis.

   4. <u>Sodium nitroprusside</u>:

      a. An older drug, long considered obsolete has recently been revived
      b. A direct peripheral vasodilator and causes marked hypotension when administered i.v.
      c. Used in acute hypertensive emergencies, not considered suitable for chronic management of hypertension.
      d. Hazardous – can precipitate marked hypotension; light sensitive. Metabolized to thiocyanate; may cause psychotic syndrome.

   5. <u>Calcium channel antagonists</u>:
      a. Being considered for monotherapy.
      b. <u>Nifedipine</u>: most potent vasodilator but also most potent <u>reflex</u> cardiac effects.
      c. Others act more directly on heart to limit reflex cardiac effects.
      d. Poor choice of drug in patients with aortic stenosis or severe heart failure.

E. <u>Inhibitor of Renin-Angiotensin System</u>

   1. <u>Captopril</u>:
      a. Inhibits the formation of angiotensin II and prevents the degradation of bradykinin.
      b. Also lowers blood pressure in "low-renin" patients.

      c. Orally effective; approved for Step I therapy; also used to treat CHF (congestive heart failure) and diagnosis of renovascular disease.

2. <u>Enalapril</u>:
      a. Action like captopril but more potent and longer acting.
      b. Prodrug; hydrolyzed in body to enalaprilate, an active metabolite.
      c. Maximum plasma levels of oral enalapril reached in 3-4 hrs; i.v. enalaprilate acts in 15 min.

3. <u>Saralasin</u>:
      a. Receptor antagonist of angiotensin II (1% of potency to stimulate receptors).
      b. Useful in the diagnosis of renin dependent hypertension.
      c. Action too short for antihypertensive therapy.

ANTICOAGULANTS

Drugs which prevent the formation of a normal blood clot (thrombus) or which suppress the extension of an existing clot. Generally most effective in the prevention of venous thrombosis.

I. Heparin:

Endogenous sulfated mucopolysaccharide found in mast cells bound to histamine and also in the liver and lungs. Physiological role is unknown.

A. Mechanism of Action:

1. Retards the conversion of prothrombin (factor II) to thrombin (principle effect)
2. Active to a lesser extent against activated forms of factors VIII, IX, X, XI and XII
3. No clinically significant effects other than the inhibition of blood clotting. Heparin causes the release of lipoprotein lipase from tissues, which hydrolyzes plasma triglycerides and has a "clearing" effect on turbid plasma.

B. Absorption, Fate and Excretion:

1. Poor oral absorption; given i.v. or s.c.
2. Duration of action; 2-4 hours
3. Dosage is adjusted according to coagulation time in therapy of acute thrombotic episodes. For prophylaxis, low doses of heparin are given which cause little change in clotting time.
4. Dosage expressed in units (1 mg is approximately 100 units)

C. Adverse Effects:

Hemorrhage, allergy, thromocytopenia, osteoporosis after long-term therapy.

D. Heparin Antagonist: Protamine sulfate

II. Oral Anticoagulants:

Coumarin (warfarin, bishydroxycoumarin) and _indanedione_ (phenindione) derivitives. Individual drugs within these chemical groups differ only in the onset and duration of action.

A. Mechanism of Action:

Antagonize the hepatic synthesis of the vitamin K-dependent clotting factors II (prothrombin), VII, IX and X. Have an onset of action of 2-3 days, during which time pre-existing levels of clotting factors are diminished. No other important physiological actions.

B. Absorption, Fate and Excretion:

1. Well absorbed orally
2. Highly bound to plasma proteins
3. Metabolized in liver prior to excretion
4. Highly variable effects from patient to patient. Adjust dosage on basis of prothrombin time.

C. Adverse Effects:

1. Hemorrhage
2. Teratogenesis, especially during first trimester
3. Liver and Kidney toxicity - seen only with indanedione derivities and limits the usefulness of this chemical class of anticoagulants.
4. Drug interactions occur among many drugs and the oral anticoagulants.

D. Oral anticoagulant antagonist: Phytonadione (vitamin K_1)

III. Thrombolytic Drugs - promote the dissolution of thrombii by stimulating the conversion of endogenous plasminogen to plasmin (fibrinolysin).

A. Streptokinase:

Produced from cultures of beta-hemolytic streptococci and is therefore antigenic, but readily available. Allergic and febrile reactions are most common non-hemorrhagic side effects.

B. Urokinase:

Obtained from human urine and not antigenic, but quite expensive.

IV. Antithrombic Drugs:

Suppress platelet function and may be useful for diseases in which platelet aggregation is thought to have an etiological role.

Aspirin	Dipyridamole
Sulfinpyrazone	Dextran

ANTI-ANEMIC DRUGS

I. Iron Deficiency Anemia

Iron is absorbed only in limited quantities from the small intestine and most of the absorption occurs in the duodenum and proximal jejunum. The drug of choice for treatment of iron deficiency anemia is <u>ferrous sulfate</u>, given 3 to 4 times per day, preferably on an empty stomach to increase iron absorption. Orally administered iron is associated with a high incidence of gastrointestinal symptoms, resulting from a direct toxic effect of iron. Patient non-compliance because of the GI symptoms is the most common cause of therapeutic failure. This problem can usually be resolved by an adjustment in dosage.

<u>Iron dextran</u> may be given by 1M or IV injection. Dosages must be carefully calculated so that the body's storage capacity is not saturated ("iron overload"). Parenterally administered iron is associated with a number of adverse effects and is indicated only when the need for iron cannot be met by oral administration.

<u>Deferoxamine mesylate</u> is a specific chelating agent for iron. It may be administered orally or parenterally for treatment of acute iron poisoning or iron overload.

II. Folic Acid Deficiency

Folic acid is widely available in the diet, and deficiency due to dietary insufficiency alone is uncommon. Alcohol and some drugs (e.g. anti-convulsants) are folate antagonists and may exacerbate megaloblastic anemia caused by folate deficiency. Folic acid is necessary for the biosynthesis of thymidylate and subsequent formation of DNA. Orally administered folic acid is usually adequate for all folate-deficient conditions.

III. Cyanocobalamin (Vitamin B_{12}) Deficiency

The daily requirement for vitamin B_{12} is extremely low (2-5 µg), and because this vitamin is found in many foods of animal origin, a deficiency due to dietary insufficiency is rare. However, the absorption of vitamin B_{12} from the gastrointestinal tract requires the prescence of a protein secreted in the stomach, intrinsic factor. The abscence of intrinsic factor, as in pernicious anemia, results in inadequate vitamin B_{12} absorption.

Vitamin B_{12} is required for the normal metabolism of folic acid, and a B_{12} deficiency will cause a megaloblastic anemia because of diminished folate-dependent DNA synthesis. However, neurological symptoms observed in pernicious anemia apparently develop from a different mechanism not involving folic acid.

Cyanocobalamin or hydroxocobalamin are normally given intramuscularly in the treatment of pernicious anemia, and treatment must be continued at monthly intervals for the rest of the patient's life. Oral vitamin B_{12} preparations with intrinsic factor derived from animals give erratic and unreliable results.

<u>REVIEW QUESTIONS</u>

<u>ONE BEST ANSWER</u>

1. _______   Changes commonly observed after digitalization of a patient with congestive heart failure may include all of the following EXCEPT:

1. An increase in myocardial contractile force
2. A marked increase in cardiac output
3. A decrease in central venous pressure
4. A decrease in blood pressure
5. A decrease in heart rate

2. _______   The usefulness of a cardiac glycoside in the management of atrial fibrillation depends upon its ability to:

1. Decrease the rate of atrial impulse formation
2. Decrease vagal control over the heart
3. Decrease conduction time through the A-V node
4. Increase the effective refractory period of the A-V node
5. Increase conduction time in the atria

3. _______   In the normal individual, digitalis can cause all of the following EXCEPT:

1. Constriction of arteriolar smooth muscle
2. Constriction of venous smooth muscle
3. Diuresis
4. Reduction of the venous return to the heart
5. Sinus tachycardia

4. _______   Cardiac glycosides are most effective in the treatment of heart failure caused by:

1. Arteriovenous fistula
2. Essential hypertension
3. Anemia
4. Thyrotoxicosis
5. Diptheria

5. _______   All of the following actions may be observed in a patient with congestive heart failure after digitalization EXCEPT:

1. Premature ventricular contractions (extrasystoles)
2. Shortening of the P-R interval of the EKG
3. Depression of the S-T segment of the EKG
4. Slowing of conduction through the A-V node
5. Inversion of the T wave of the EKG

<u>ONE BEST ANSWER</u>

6. _______ All of the following are associated with the actions or side effects of procainamide EXCEPT:

1. The amide linkage in the molecule prevents rapid hydrolysis by plasma esterases
2. It decreases membrane responsiveness
3. Overdosage may stimulate the CNS and cause convulsions
4. It increases blood pressure
5. Chronic administration may cause blood dyscrasias

7. _______ All of the following are associated with the actions or side effects of quinidine EXCEPT:

1. It may cause sinus tachycardia because of its anti-cholinergic action
2. It may cause an increase in ventricular rate (paradoxical tachycardia)
3. It may cause ventricular fibrillation in toxic doses
4. It may increase the automaticity of ectopic ventricular pacemaker cells
5. It may decrease myocardial contractility

8. _______ Which statement is true with respect to lidocaine given in therapeutic concentrations?

1. It depresses normal ventricular conduction
2. It delays A-V conduction
3. It depresses ventricular automaticity
4. It prolongs the P-R interval
5. It prolongs the QRS interval

9. _______ Coronary blood flow, myocardial contractility and oxygen consumption are augmented by all of the following agents EXCEPT:

1. Nicotine
2. Theophylline
3. Isoproterenol
4. Amyl nitrite

10. _______ All of the following effects are caused by nitroglycerin EXCEPT:

1. Postural hypotension and syncope
2. Methemoglobinemia
3. Contraction of the sphincter of Oddi
4. Tachycardia
5. Reduction of myocardial oxygen consumption

<u>ONE BEST ANSWER</u>

11. _______   The most efficacious of all diuretics that have sulfamyl groups is:

1. Chlorothiazide
2. Hydrochlorothiazide
3. Furosemide
4. Ethacrynic acid

12. _______   Prolonged administration of chlorothiazide is likely to result in:

1. Hyperchloremic acidosis
2. Hyperkalemic acidosis
3. Hypochloremic, hypokalemic alkalosis
4. Metabolic acidosis (low K+ and HCO_3^-)
5. Respiratory alkalosis

13. _______   The anticoagulant action of bishydroxycoumarin can be effectively counteracted by:

1. Vitamin C
2. Vitamin K
3. Thromboplastin
4. EDTA
5. Phenindione

14. _______   All of the following are true of lidocaine EXCEPT:

1. Decreases ventricular automaticity
2. May cause convulsions in overdosage
3. May cause hypotension
4. Oral administration on a chronic basis may prevent the reoccurrence of paroxysmal atrial tachycardia
5. Is useful in the emergency treatment of ventricular arrhythmias after myocardial infarction

15. _______   Therapeutic concentrations of quinidine may cause all of the following EXCEPT:

1. Decrease in the effect of vagus nerve stimulation on the heart
2. Decrease in myocardial contractility
3. Decrease in the rate of rise of the upstroke of the action potential (phase O)
4. Decrease in membrane responsiveness
5. Decrease in the Q-T interval of the electrocardiogram

16. _______   Slow diastolic (phase 4) depolarization of automatic cells is decreased by all of the following EXCEPT:

1. Acetylcholine
2. Quinidine
3. Bretyllium
4. Hyperkalemia
5. Phenytoin

<u>ONE BEST ANSWER</u>

17. _______ Automaticity refers to:

    1. The speed of a single cardiac contraction
    2. The rate of depolarization of atrial muscle
    3. The rate of repolarization of ventricular muscle
    4. The rate of conduction in the A-V node
    5. The frequency of discharge of a pacemaker area in the heart

18. _______ All of the following statements are correct in regard to cardiac
arrhythmias EXCEPT:

    1. Paroxysmal atrial tachycardia without A-V block may occur in
       otherwise healthy patients
    2. Paroxysmal atrial tachycardia with A-V block is usually due to
       digitalis intoxication
    3. Ventricular tachycardia is usually more grave in prognosis than
       atrial tachycardia
    4. Cardiac arrhythmias due to digitalis intoxication are effectively
       treated with KCl, phenytoin and/or lidocaine
    5. Propranolol is indicated for the treatment of congestive heart
       failure due to cardiac arrhythmias

19. _______ Which one of the following mechanisms best explains the
antihypertensive actions of clonidine?

    1. Blockade of B_1-adrenergic receptors
    2. Blockade of CNS <u>alpha</u>-adrenergic receptors
    3. Stimulation of CNS <u>alpha</u>-adrenergic receptors
    4. Blockade of peripheral <u>alpha</u>-adrenergic receptors
    5. Stimulation of peripheral <u>alpha</u>-adrenergic receptors

20. _______ A syndrome resembling systemic lupus erythematosus occurs in about
10% of patients receiving moderate to high doses of which one of the
following antihypertensive drugs?

    1. Hydralazine
    2. Hydrochlorothiazide
    3. Diazoxide
    4. Sodium nitroprusside
    5. Guanethidine

21. _______ Which one of the following would most likely increase plasma renin
activity?

    1. Blood transfusion
    2. <u>Alpha</u>-methyldopa
    3. Propranolol
    4. Chlorothiazide
    5. Metaprolol

<u>ONE BEST ANSWER</u>

22. _______ Which of the following drugs is of clinical interest because of its
ability to inhibit platelet aggregation?

    1. Streptokinase
    2. Bishydroxycoumarin
    3. Dipyridamole
    4. Propranolol
    5. Aminocaproic acid

23. _______ Drug of choice for treatment of diabetes insipidus of pituitary
origin:

    1. Vasopressin injection (i.v.)
    2. Clofibrate
    3. Chlorothiazide
    4. Desmopressin
    5. Lypressin

24. _______ Drug of choice for the treatment of nephrogenic diabetes insipidus:

    1. Lithium carbonate
    2. Chlorpropamide
    3. Chlorothiazide
    4. Desmopressin
    5. Vasopressin tannate injection (i.m.)

<u>MULTIPLE TRUE-FALSE</u>
Directions: For each of the statements below, <u>ONE</u> or <u>MORE</u> of the completions
given is correct.

    1 - If only 1, 2 and 3 are correct
    2 - If only 1 and 3 are correct
    3 - If only 2 and 4 are correct
    4 - If only 4 is correct
    5 - If all are correct

25. _______ Clofibrate:

    1. Is an ion exchange resin
    2. Drug of choice for type III hyperlipidemia
    3. Has no effect on triglycerides but markedly lowers cholesterol
    4. Skeletal muscle weakness causes

<u>MULTIPLE TRUE-FALSE</u>
<u>Directions Summarized:</u>

1	2	3	4	5
1,2,3	1,3	2,4	4	all are
only	only	only	only	correct

26. _______ Diazoxide:

1. Is a potent diuretic agent
2. Produces a marked hypoglycemia in non-diabetic patients
3. Increase blood pressure
4. Is a thiazide analogue

27. _______ Furosemide:

1. Increases blood flow in the <u>vasa recta</u>
2. Produces diuresis in the dehydrated patient
3. Induces severe hypokalemia
4. Inhibits sodium reabsorption mainly in proximal tubules

28. _______ Acetazolamide:

1. Is a carbonic anhydrase inhibitor
2. Produces an acid urine
3. Increases ammonia concentration in renal vein blood
4. Increases urinary ammonium excretion

29. _______ Triamterene:

1. Increases plasma potassium concentration
2. Inhibits sodium reabsorption in the distal tubule
3. Used with thiazide diuretics
4. Antagonizes competitively the action of aldosterone on renal
   tubules

30. _______ Potent diuretics generally:

1. Increase magnesium excretion in the urine
2. Enhance sodium excretion in the urine
3. Increase aldosterone secretion as a compensatory mechanism
4. In excessive doses, cause dehydration and orthostatic hypotension

31. _______ Mercurial diuretics:

1. May be given to edematous patients with glomerulonephritis
2. Are less potent in the presence of systemic alkalosis
3. Tend to produce hyperchloremic acidosis
4. Have a strong affinity for the sulfhydryl (SH) groups on enzymes
   in renal tubules

<u>MULTIPLE TRUE-FALSE</u>
<u>Directions Summarized:</u>

1	2	3	4	5
1,2,3	1,3	2,4	4	all are
only	only	only	only	correct

32. _______ Warfarin:

    1. Has a slow onset of action
    2. Is given orally or by injection
    3. Has a long duration of action
    4. Interferes with the synthesis of prothrombin in the liver

33. _______ Heparin:

    1. Is most often given intravenously
    2. Is the strongest organic acid naturally occurring in the body
    3. Lowers plasma lipid levels
    4. Is metabolized by a liver enzyme

34. _______ Organic nitrites can:

    1. Relax vascular smooth muscle
    2. Cause fainting as a result of vascular pooling of blood
    3. Cause methemoglobinemia
    4. Cause a reflex increase in heart rate

35. _______ Nitroglycerin:

    1. Can relieve the pain of angina pectoris
    2. Has a rapid onset of action
    3. Is rapidly absorbed sublingually
    4. Has a long duration of action

36. _______ Cardiac glycosides toxicity is enhanced by:

    1. Decreased extracellular Ca^{++}
    2. Decreased stimulation rate
    3. Increased extracellular Mg^{++}
    4. Decreased extracellular K^{+}

37. _______ Conduction velocity in a reentry arrhythmia path may be influenced
        by:

    1. Membrane potential just prior to stimulation or excitation
    2. Action potential duration
    3. Anatomy/structure/mass of the conducting pathway
    4. Inward (depolarizing) current magnitude

<u>MULTIPLE TRUE-FALSE</u>
<u>Directions Summarized:</u>

1	2	3	4	5
1,2,3	1,3	2,4	4	all are
only	only	only	only	correct

38. _______ Cardiac conduction properties always required for reentry type
arrhythmias are:

    1. Impulse conduction velocity slower than seen in normal
       ventricular muscle
    2. Bidirectional conduction block
    3. Unidirectional conduction block
    4. Impulse conduction velocity faster than seen in normal
       ventricular muscle

39. _______ Which of the following can be used rationally to augment cardiac
glycoside therapy of congestive heart failure?

    1. Vasodilators to decrease afterload
    2. Treat the underlying cause for heart failure
    3. Diuretics to help decrease edema and volume overload
    4. Raise serum K^+ to extend therapeutic range of the glycoside

40. _______ Which of the following decrease cardiac work?

    1. Nitroglycerin
    2. Hydralazine
    3. Verapamil
    4. Catecholamines

41. _______ Rate of firing of an automatic (pacemaker) foci may be decreased by:

    1. Increasing (more negative) the maximum diastolic potential
    2. Increasing the rate of phase 4 depolarization
    3. Increasing the action potential duration
    4. Increasing (more negative) the threshold potential for excitation

42. _______ Depresses conduction velocity of the <u>normal</u> myocardium at therapeutic
concentrations:

    1. Lidocaine
    2. Bretyllium
    3. Phenytoin
    4. Quinidine

<u>MULTIPLE TRUE-FALSE</u>
Directions Summarized:

1	2	3	4	5
1,2,3	1,3	2,4	4	all are
only	only	only	only	correct

43. _______ Heparin:

1. Decreases absorption of vitamin K from the gut
2. Is an effective anticoagulant for freshly-drawn blood
3. Is enhanced in its effectiveness by the concurrent administration of phenobarbital
4. Can be antagonized <u>in vivo</u> by the administration of protamine sulfate

44. _______ Warfarin:

1. Is not useful as an anticoagulant for freshly-drawn blood
2. Overdose is treated by withholding the drug and administration of vitamin K
3. Is contraindicated in patients with potential bleeding problems, i.e., patients with malignant hypertension or active tuberculosis
4. Is immediately effective after intravenous administration

45. _______ Drug interactions which adversely affect the therapy with orally effective anticoagulant agents might occur by:

1. Their displacement from binding sites on plasma protein
2. An increase in their metabolism
3. A decrease in their metabolism
4. Elimination of enteric bacteria by non-absorbed antibiotic agents

46. _______ Iron containing preparations:

1. Are indicated in the treatment of megaloblastic anemias
2. Taken in excessive amounts by children can cause gastric necrosis, cardiovascular shock and death
3. Are absorbed primarily in the ferric form
4. Are stored in substantial amounts in the reticuloendothelial cells of the liver and spleen

47. _______ Thrombolytic drugs:

1. Urokinase
2. Aminocaproic acid
3. Streptokinase
4. Sulfinpyrazone

<u>MULTIPLE TRUE-FALSE</u>
<u>Directions Summarized:</u>

1	2	3	4	5
1,2,3	1,3	2,4	4	all are
only	only	only	only	correct

48. _______ Which of the following statements are true of pernicious anemia?

  1. The megaloblastic anemia is likely to improve if high doses of folic acid are taken
  2. Neurological symptoms are likely to improve if high doses of folic acid are taken
  3. Therapy is initiated with daily injections of cyanocobalamine to replete hepatic stores of the vitamin
  4. Long-term therapy consists of daily oral cyanocobalamin plus multivitamin supplements for the rest of the patient's life

<u>MATCHING</u>

Match the following drugs with the most appropriate side effects. (<u>Use each answer only once</u>)

  1. Minoxidil
  2. Reserpine
  3. Hydralazine
  4. Diazoxide
  5. Pargyline

49. _______ Lupus-like syndrome

50. _______ Hyperglycemia

51. _______ Hypertrichosis

52. _______ Sedation and increased G.I. motility

53. _______ Hypertensive crisis possible with tyramine intake

<u>MATCHING</u>

<u>Use only once</u>

1. Prazosin
2. Pindolol
3. Nadolol
4. Atenolol
5. Metaprolol
6. Labetalol

54. _______ Once per day administration due to long half-life

55. _______ Intrinsic sympathomimetic activity

56. _______ "Cardioselective", mainly renal elimination

57. _______ "Cardioselective", mainly hepatic elimination

58. _______ <u>Alpha</u> and <u>beta</u> blockade

59. _______ <u>Alpha</u>-1 adrenoceptor selective

* * * * * * * * * *

1. Digoxin
2. Quinidine
3. Both
4. Neither

60. _______ In toxic concentrations, specifically inhibits the
sodium-potassium-dependent ATP-ase

61. _______ Toxic signs are partially antagonized by increasing extracellular
potassium ion concentration

62. _______ Causes a variety of allergic, hypersensitivity reactions

63. _______ Causes hypotension, particularly when administered I.V.

64. _______ Often used for long term therapy

65. _______ Effective orally in the management of certain cardiac arrhythmias

66. _______ In therapeutic (non-toxic) concentrations decreases the rate of rise
of the action potential from Purkinje fibers

67. _______ Contraindicated in asthmatic patients

68. _______ The drug can kill by causing ventricular fibrillation

<u>MATCHING</u>

    1.   Procainamide
    2.   Disopyramide
    3.   Propranolol
    4.   Phenytoin
    5.   Verapamil

69. _______ Orally effective group II antiarrhythmic agent (lidocaine type)

70. _______ Systemic lupus erythematosis-like syndrome is associated with the use of this agent

71. _______ Slow inward current (Ca^{++}) channel blocking agent

72. _______ Orally effective group I antiarrhythmic agent with high anticholinergic activity and propensity to cause heart failure in compromised patients

73. _______ Useful for the treatment of angina pectoris and cardiac arrhythmias

* * * * * * * * * *

    1.   Digoxin
    2.   Digitoxin
    3.   Both
    4.   Neither

74. _______ Excreted primarily via the kidney

75. _______ Toxicity increased by high Ca^{++}

76. _______ Choice in presence of severe kidney failure

77. _______ Half-life of 5-7 days

78. _______ Enhances conduction in the A-V node

79. _______ Dangerous in combination with quinidine

80. _______ Most rapidly acting of the cardiac glycosides

<u>MATCHING</u>

Choose the one most appropriate response – use each choice only once.

1. Mercaptomerin
2. Acetazolamide
3. Chlorothiazide
4. Ethacrynic acid
5. Spironolactone
6. Mannitol
7. Triamterene
8. Theophylline

81. _______ Diuresis with decreased potassium loss due to aldosterone antagonism

82. _______ Ototoxicity is a serious complication associated with this drug

83. _______ Hypochloremic alkalosis leads to a decrease in the diuretic effectiveness of this agent with time

84. _______ Metabolic acidosis leads to a decrease in the diuretic effectiveness of this agent

85. _______ Often used to decrease potassium loss in conjunction with other diuretics (eg., thiazides). When used alone may cause hyperkalemia

86. _______ Used in treatment of diabetes insipidus and hypertension

87. _______ Useful in preventing renal failure in very low renal perfusion states where other agents may fail, contraindicated in cardiac decompensation

88. _______ Diuresis may be a side effect of respiratory therapy with this methylxanthine

ANSWERS

1.   **4**   Blood pressure in a patient with congestive failure is usually about normal or a bit on the low side, depending upon the severity of the failure and the degree of compensation. Digitalis, because of the improved cardiac output, will improve hemodynamics and return pressure towards normal; it definitely will not fall.

2.   **4**   When effective refractory period is prolonged, fewer impulses can pass through the node and ventricular rate is slowed.

3.   **5**   Digitalis enhances vagal tone to the sinus node by several mechanisms and will slow the discharge of impulses from the node. Thus, sinus bradycardia is the result unless vagal tone is already high; in this case, heart rate may not change.

4.   **2**   Glycosides are most effective in low output failure; they are ineffective in high output failure or if myocardial damage results from a toxic process.

5.   **2**   Glycosides enhance vagal tone to the AV node to slow conduction of impulses through the node. The P-R interval is an index of AV conduction time. Since AV conduction time is longer, P-R interval is prolonged.

6.   **4**   Procainamide directly relaxes vascular smooth muscle to cause hypotension.

7.   **4**   Quinidine slows diastolic depolarization (rate of rise of phase 4 of the action potential - the prepotential) of all automatic cells. This is the mechanism by which quinidine decreases automaticity.

8.   **3**   Lidocaine and other anti-arrhythmic drugs decrease automaticity by the same mechanism (explained in #7 for quinidine).

9.   **4**   All except amyl nitrite are considered "malignant" vasodilators; they stimulate the heart causing increase in work load and a relative hypoxia; the hypoxia stimulates the blood vessels to dilate. Amyl nitrite decreases work load because of direct vasodilator effect on all vascular smooth muscle; decreased work load on the heart leads to decreased oxygen demand.

10.   **3**   Nitroglycerin relaxes all types of smooth muscle - bronchioles, GI, GU, biliary tree, etc. NG relieves pain of cholecystitis and biliary colic.

11.   **3**   Furosemide is a "high ceiling" or "loop diuretic" and is a sulfonamide derivative.

12.   **3**   Promotes urinary excretion of chloride and potassium leading to hypochloremia and hypokalemia; the hypokalemic state (potassium depletion) leads to alkalosis.

13.   **2**

14.   **4**   Lidocaine is not effective orally; also not very effective in atrial arrhythmias

15.   **5**   Prolongs Q-T interval by increasing action potential duration

16.   **3**

17.   **5**   The physiological definition of automaticity

18.   **5**   Propranolol decreases contractility and would aggravate failure

19.   **3**

20.   **1**

21.   4   Plasma renin levels would increase in response to decreased perfusion pressure of kidney, decreased sympathetic tone or due to Na^+ loss. Alpha-methyldopa would decrease sympathetic tone to kidney thus inhibit neural renin release. The <u>beta</u> blockers would block the renal receptors activated by sympathetic tone to kidney.

22.   3

23.   4

24.   3

25.   3

26.   4

27.   1

28.   2

29.   1

30.   5

31.   3

32.   5

33.   5

34.   5

35.   1

36.   4

37.   5   The conduction velocity is directly proportional to the depolarizing current magnitude. This may be directly influenced by the tissue mass and indirectly by the potential prior to excitation (sodium current inactivation or reactivation). The action potential duration will only affect the conduction velocity of a premature beat falling on the repolarization phase of the action potential by a change in potential just prior to excitation.

38.   2   Slow conduction is required for the reentering impulse to arrive at the point of reentry after the end of the effective refractory period. Unidirectional block is an absolute requirement. See any discussion of reentry arrhythmias.

39.   1   The therapeutic and toxic effects of cardiac glycosides are closely linked to extracellular potassium. Although toxicity would be decreased by raising serum K^+, the therapeutic effect also would be decreased.

40.   1

41.   2   Answer 1 is true because an increase in potential difference between maximum diastolic potential and threshold will require a longer time to reach threshold. Answer 4 is false for the opposite reason. The rate or speed of depolarization is directly proportional to firing rate and increasing action potential duration with no other changes will decrease frequency of firing.

42.   4

43.   3

44.   1

45.   5

46.   3

47.   2   Aminocaproic acid is an inhibitor of plasmin and plasminogen activator, and antagonizes the actions of streptokinase and urokinase. Sulfinpyrazone is a uricosuric drug with anti-platelet activity.

48.   __2__   Vitamin B_{12} is necessary for a demethylation reaction of dietary folic acid, which allows the folate to function in DNA synthesis. During vitamin B_{12} deficiency, folic acid supplementation will allow delivery of some folate to the bone marrow in a metabolically active form, so improvement of the anemia is likely to occur. The neurological symptoms of pernicious anemia are apparently related to the B_{12} deficiency, and will not respond to folate therapy. Vitamin B_{12} is not absorbed effectively in pernicious anemia, due to inavailability of intrinsic factor, so that oral cyanocobalamin is not likely to be effective.

49.   __3__
50.   __4__
51.   __1__
52.   __2__
53.   __5__
54.   __3__
55.   __2__
56.   __4__
57.   __5__
58.   __6__
59.   __1__
60.   __1__
61.   __1__
62.   __2__
63.   __2__
64.   __3__
65.   __3__
66.   __2__
67.   __4__
68.   __3__
69.   __4__
70.   __1__
71.   __5__
72.   __2__
73.   __3__
74.   __1__
75.   __3__
76.   __2__
77.   __2__
78.   __4__
79.   __3__
80.   __4__
81.   __5__
82.   __4__
83.   __1__
84.   __2__
85.   __7__
86.   __3__
87.   __6__
88.   __8__

SECTION VI: <u>ENDOCRINES</u>

THYROID - ANTITHYROID

<u>DRUGS USED IN TREATMENT OF THYROID DISORDERS</u>

A. Hyperthyroidism

    1. Inhibitors of hormone synthesis
        a. Propylthiouracil and methimazole (methimazole is more potent and has a
            longer duration than PTU)
        b. Inhibit oxidation of I^- to I_2
        c. Block coupling of iodotyrosines
        d. Cross placenta and excreted into milk; PTU transfers less than
            methimazole
        e. May produce remission, but relapse occurs frequently
        f. Agranulocytosis is the most serious untoward reaction; rash, the most
            common

    2. Iodide (Lugol's solution, Strong iodine solution)
        a. Large doses produce temporary remission; used before surgery to
            decrease vascularity and in thyrotoxic crisis
        b. Inhibits hormone release; inhibits iodide transport and hormone
            synthesis
        c. Effect is not sustained

    3. Radioiodine
        a. Destroys tissue
        b. Used as an alternative to surgery, especially in older patients and
            those with heart disease
        c. High incidence of subsequent hypothyroidism

    4. Propranolol
        a. Controls some symptoms
        b. Mechanism of action unclear, may be anti-adrenergic effect, may be
            inhibition of T_4 conversion to T_3

B. Hypothyroidism

    1. Drugs used are glandular extracts, (thyroid, thyroglobulin), pure
        hormones, (levothyroxine, liothyronine) or mixtures of T_4 and T_3 (liotrix)
    2. Levothyroxine is drug of choice
    3. T_4 has a slower onset, is more extensively bound to plasma proteins and
        has a longer duration than T_3
    4. Uses
        a. Myxedema and less severe deficiencies
        b. Simple goiter to suppress TSH
        c. Not recommended for weight reduction, reproductive disorders, or
            depression

ADRENOCORTICAL STEROIDS

A. Glucocorticoids

1. Natural – hydrocortisone (cortisol); some salt retention

2. Synthetic – effective orally, parenterally, topically
    a. Short acting (significant salt retention)
            Hydrocortisone
    b. Intermediate-acting
            Prednisone
            Methylprednisolone
            Triamcinolone
    c. Long-acting
            Dexamethasone
            Betamethasone

3. Effects
    a. Metabolic – hyperglycemia, lipolysis, protein catabolism
    b. Anti-inflammatory – inhibit every step of inflammatory process;
        inhibit neutrophil actions, eicosanoid release, late-phase allergic
        reactions
    c. Immunosuppressive
    d. Permissive – "necessary but not sufficient" role in concert with other
        hormones or regulatory forces

4. Uses
    a. Treat adrenocortical insufficiency – supplement with salt-retaining
        hormone
    b. In congenital adrenal hyperplasia to suppress ACTH
    c. Therapy of non-endocrine diseases
        1) Secondary agent in rheumatoid arthritis
        2) Leukemia, lymphoma
        3) Severe allergic reactions
        4) Asthma
        5) Cerebral edema

5. Major untoward effects
    a. Large doses for less than 1 week little problem
    b. Long periods – resemble patient with Cushing's syndrome
    c. Suppression of HPA axis
    d. Metabolic
        1) Weight gain, Cushing's habitus
        2) Hyperglycemia and diabetes
        3) Osteoporosis
        4) Muscle wasting
    e. Gastric ulcer
    f. Psychosis
    g. Cataracts and glaucoma
    h. Increased susceptibility to infection

6. Dosage schedules
    a. Topical application produces little systemic effect
    b. High doses used daily to achieve desired effect, then switch to
        alternate day therapy

      c. To suppress ACTH, use daily small doses or slowly absorbed preparations given parenterally

B. Mineralocorticoids

    1. Aldosterone, fludrocortisone
      a. Latter may be used in adrenal insufficiency for salt retaining function

C. Inhibitors of adrenal hormone synthesis

    1. Mitotane – produces adrenal atrophy and used in carcinoma of gland
    2. Aminoglutethimide – blocks conversion of cholesterol to pregnenolone, used in adrenal carcinoma
    3. Metyrapone – used to assess ACTH secretion by blocking cortisol synthesis (inhibits 11-hydroxylation)
    4. Trilostane – inhibits 3 beta-hydroxysteroid dehydrogenase, used in Cushing's syndrome, adrenal cancer

PARATHRYOID HORMONE

A. Maintains blood calcium by

    1. Affecting mobilization of bone calcium
    2. Affecting absorption of calcium by gut
    3. Affecting excretion of calcium by kidney
    4. Increasing formation of active vitamin D3 by kidney

B. PTH not used often therapeutically because same effect obtained with large doses of vitamin D.

C. Hypercalcemia

    1. Treatment symptomatic by forcing fluids, removing tumor
    2. Calcitonin has been tried but with limited success because of tolerance development

INSULIN

A. Used in treatment of insulin-dependent diabetic patients (IDDM) and some
    individuals with noninsulin-dependent diabetes

B. Preparations made from beef or pork pancreas, or semisynthetic and synthetic
    human insulin. They vary in duration of action because of:
    1. Insoluble protein added - protamine zinc or NPH
    2. Crystal size - lente series

C. Insulin controls hyperglycemia and ketoacid formation by several mechanisms
    including:
    1. Increased transport of glucose into fat and muscle, glycogen synthesis
    2. Inhibition of lipolysis, increased triglyceride synthesis
    3. Inhibition of protein catabolism, increased amino acid transport
    4. Decreased hepatic glucose production, glycogen synthesis
    5. Decreased glucagon secretion

D. Insulin therapy may have no effect on cardiovascular lesion associated with
    chronic insulin deficiency

E. Untoward reactions
    1. Hypoglycemia
        a. Wrong dose
        b. Unusual exercise
        c. Not eating at regular time
        d. Treat with i.v. glucose
        e. Patients can be instructed in the use of glucagon for treating
            reactions
    2. Allergic reactions and localized atrophy less common with newer single
        component insulin preparations

F. Insulin antagonists
    1. Glucocorticoids
    2. Pregnancy and birth control pills
    3. Weight gain
    4. Infections
    5. Surgical procedures

G. Treatment of ketoacidosis includes:
    1. I.V. insulin
    2. Hypotonic saline - need to replenish and maintain intravascular volume
    3. Sometimes bicarbonate - only if pH is below 7.0
    4. Sometimes KCl - more often than not; whole body potassium low even with
        normokalemia
    5. Sometimes phosphate - only if hypophosphatemic
    6. Get glucose below 250 mg%, but not too rapidly in order to avoid cerebral
        edema

H. Oral hypoglycemic agents
    1. May increase incidence of cardiovascular deaths (UGDP study); but
        conclusions of study in dispute
    2. Sulfonylurea derivatives (tolbutamide, chlorpropamide, glipizide,
        glyburide and others)
        a. Mechanism of action

1. Releases insulin from pancreas
2. Might also have effects on liver. Mechanism uncertain: cyclic-AMP, calcium, or increased sensitivity to glucose
3. Increases number of insulin receptors on cells
4. Decreases gluconeogenesis

b. Differences in duration between derivatives depends on rate of metabolism by the liver and type of metabolites; i.e., active or inactive Chlorpropamide metabolized slowest ($t\frac{1}{2}$ 36 hr)

c. Can interact with other drugs by:
1. Protein binding displacement
2. Changes in microsomal drug metabolism
3. Decreased renal excretion of active metabolites
4. Additive effects of glucose disposition (i.e., aspirin)
5. Ethanol may increase or decrease hypoglycemic action; Disulfiram-like effect possible

d. Useful only in non-insulin requiring diabetics, failure of therapy with continued use occurs (secondary failure)

e. Adverse reactions
1. Hypoglycemia
2. Granulocytopenia
3. Cholestatic jaundice
4. Allergic reactions
5. Chlorpropamide may cause water retention because of augmentation of ADH action

3. Phenformin – not currently available in U.S. except by special request of FDA
a. Differences from sulfonylureas:
1. Does not release insulin
2. Does not produce hypoglycemia
b. Mechanism of action
1. Increases glycolysis
2. Decreases gluconeogenesis
3. Decreases glucose absorption from GI tract
c. Adverse reactions
1. Nausea and vomiting
2. Anorexia
3. Lactic acidosis
d. Is not used therapeutically because of tendency to produce lactic acidosis

OVARIAN HORMONES AND OVULATORY AGENTS

A. Estrogens

1. Preparations

a. Steroids
1. Natural – estradiol and various esters of estradiol, parenteral; conjugated estrogens – oral, parenteral or topical
2. Synthetic – ethinyl estradiol, mestranol – both oral
b. Non-steroid
1. Diethylstilbesterol and related compounds
2. Can be taken orally or parenterally
c. Route of administration depends on whether metabolized by liver

2. Uses

    a. Replacement therapy – non-development of ovaries, castration, menopause (give cyclically with progestin unless uterus removed)
    b. Osteoporosis
    c. Dysmenorrhea (with progestin)
    d. Contraception
    e. Acne
    f. Cancer

3. Adverse effects

    a. Nausea
    b. Breast tenderness
    c. Weight gain
    d. Increased skin pigmentation
    e. Thrombophlebitis, thromboembolism
    f. Cancer
    g. Benign hepatoma

B. Progestins

1. Preparations
    a. Natural – progesterone and various esters, parenteral
    b. Synthetic – norethindrone, ethynodiol, medroxyprogesterone, norgestrel; oral (may have estrogenic or adrenogenic effects, as well

2. Uses
    a. Contraception
    b. Dysmenorrhea, endometriosis-suppresses ovulation and subsequent uterine changes (used with estrogen)
    c. Dysfunctional uterine bleeding
    d. Endometrial carcinoma

3. Adverse reactions
    a. Cholestatic jaundice

C. Hormonal Contraception

1. Oral contraceptives
    a. Estrogen + progestin combination
    b. Progestins alone

2. Action
    a. Inhibit ovulation
    b. Act on uterus to decrease conception and implantation by changing secretions and motility

3. Adverse reactions
    a. Mild
        1. Nausea, breast tenderness, edema, all of these estrogen-dependent
        2. Serum proteins – foul-up thyroid, adrenal and pituitary tests. Fibrinogen increased
        3. Increased skin pigmentation
        4. Diabetic glucose tolerance curves

```
        5.  Break-through bleeding
        6.  Vaginal infections
     b.  Severe
        1.  Jaundice
        2.  Thrombophlebitis, thromboembolism
        3.  Hypertension
```

D. Ovulatory agents

```
  1.  Clomiphene
     a.  Antiestrogen with weak estrogenic activity
     b.  Acts by binding estrogen receptors and preventing the normal "feedback
         inhibition" by estrogen in the hypothalamus and pituitary; increases
         GnRH and gonadotropin secretion
     c.  Used in anovulatory states
     d.  Adverse reactions
        1.  Mild menopausal symptoms
        2.  Ovarian cyst formation
        3.  Multiple births

  2.  Human menopausal gonadotropin
     a.  Made from urine of post-menopausal women; contains both FSH and LH
     b.  Used with chorionic gonadotropin, which resembles LH in structure and
         function, to induce ovulation
     c.  Used in males with HCG to stimulate spermatogenesis
     d.  Adverse reactions
        1.  Multiple births
        2.  Ovarian enlargement with possible pain and ascites
```

ANDROGENS AND ANABOLIC STEROIDS

A. Agents

```
  1.  Natural-testosterone and esters; most given i.m.; most effective for full
      replacement therapy
  2.  Derivatives of testosterone - methyltestosterone, fluoxymesterone,
      danazol, oxymetholone; orally active, 17-alkyl substituted
```

B. Uses

```
  1.  Hypogonadism - delayed puberty
  2.  Hypopituitarism - to promote growth at puberty; must be careful of
      epiphyseal closure
  3.  Promotion of anabolism to reverse protein loss with severe disease
  4.  Anemias - to stimulate erythropoiesis; large doses and prolonged treatment
      are required
  5.  Mammary carcinoma
  6.  Endometriosis (danazol)
  7.  Hereditary angioneurotic edema (17-alkyl androgens)
```

C. Adverse reactions

```
  1.  Masculinization (acne, facial hair, deepening of voice are earliest
      effects)
  2.  Can produce increased libido, priapism
```

3. Sodium retention and edema
4. Given to pregnant women may masculinize fetus
5. 17-alkyl substituted derivatives impair liver function and cause cholestatic jaundice
6. Do not give with carcinoma of prostate
7. Liver carcinoma
8. Impotence and azoospermia
9. Feminization (gynecomastia)

D. Antiandrogen - cyproterone acetate

ANTERIOR PITUITARY

A. Growth hormone

Somatrem - purified polypeptide of recombinant DNA orgin, identical to human GH plus an additional amino acid, methionine

B. ACTH

1. Natural - provided in insoluble preparations to increase duration
2. Synthetic cosyntropin. First 24 amino acids of β-ACTH
3. Uses
   a. Too short acting for most treatments
   b. Test for adrenal insufficiency
   c. Test for adrenal carcinoma

C. FSH and LH - use HCG or HMG

D. TSH

1. Preparation for I.M. use
2. Uses
   a. To increase ^{131}I uptake
   b. Diagnosis of pituitary insufficiency
3. Adverse reactions
   a. Do not use in patients with severe cardiovascular disease
   b. Allergic reactions

POSTERIOR PITUITARY HORMONES

A. Vasopressin (Antidiuretic Hormone) (See Section V for further discussion)

B. Oxytocin

1. Both hormones are synthesized in the hypothalmus, and are transported to the posterior pituitary where they are stored
2. Both are peptide hormones consisting of 9 amino acids, and they differ only in the amino acids at positions 3 and 8
3. Both have a short half-life (15-30 min)
4. Because of their chemical similarities, vasopressin has slight oxytocic activity, and oxytocin has slight antidiuretic activity. However, oxytocin has no vasoconstricting activity

REVIEW QUESTIONS

<u>ONE BEST ANSWER</u>

1. _______ The symptoms of hypothyroidism can be controlled with adequate doses
of:

   1. Thyroxine
   2. Tri-iodothyronine
   3. Desiccated thyroid powder
   4. All of the above
   5. None of the above

2. _______ Propylthiouracil decreases the secretion of thyroxine by:

   1. Inhibiting the uptake of iodide by the thyroid gland
   2. Interfering with the secretion of TSH by the pituitary
   3. Interfering with the organic binding of iodine
   4. None of the above

3. _______ All of the following are actions of insulin <u>EXCEPT</u>:

   1. Decreased mobilization of free fatty acids
   2. Increased uptake of glucose by muscle
   3. Increased rate of gluconeogenesis
   4. Increased formation of glycerophosphate by fat cells

4. _______ Large doses of Vitamin D can be used in the treatment of
hypoparathyroidism because:

   1. It increases the mobilization of calcium from bone
   2. It decreases the excretion of calcium by the kidney
   3. It enhances the absorption of calcium from the gastrointestinal
      tract
   4. All of the above

5. _______ Clomiphene has been used in women for the treatment of infertility
because:

   1. It increases the secretion of FSH and LH by competing with
      estrogen for inhibitory sites in the hypothalamus
   2. It is structurally related to diethylstilbesterol
   3. It increases the chance that a fertilized ovum will be implanted
   4. It increases the libido in ovulating women

6. _______ Patients taking large doses of glucocorticoids should not abruptly
stop taking the drug because:

   1. A rebound hyperglycemia may result in persistent diabetes
   2. Latent infections such as tuberculosis may become active
   3. Rapid mobilization of calcium from bone will occur
   4. Signs of adrenal failure may be seen due to suppression of ACTH
      secretion during treatment with resultant adrenal atrophy

<u>ONE BEST ANSWER</u>

7. _______ Severe adverse reactions are a therapeutic problem in the use of adrenal glucocorticoids in all but one of the following conditions. That one is:

    1. Suppression of the inflammatory reaction in collagen diseases
    2. Treatment of acute and chronic lymphocytic leukemias
    3. Acute treatment of anaphylactic shock
    4. Treatment of severe chronic bronchial asthma

8. _______ Dexamethasone produces all of the following metabolic changes EXCEPT:

    1. Increase in hepatic glycogen storage
    2. Hyperglycemia
    3. Decrease in protein synthesis in lymphocytes
    4. Redistribution of fat in the body
    5. Decrease in gluconeogenesis

9. _______ All of the following would be favorably affected by treatment with estrogens EXCEPT:

    1. Menopause
    2. Failure of ovarian development
    3. Postpartum bleeding
    4. Acne

10. _______ All of the following states might result from severe insulin deficiency <u>EXCEPT</u>:

    1. Loss of cellular potassium
    2. Metabolic acidosis
    3. Increased 2, 3-diphosphoglycerate in red blood cells
    4. Decreased vascular volume
    5. Increased cellular content of sorbitol

11. _______ Which one of the following is true of the complex of protamine with insulin?

    1. The complex is readily soluble and can be given I.V. to treat diabetic coma
    2. The complex has effects qualitatively different from those of regular insulin
    3. The complex may be used whenever a prolonged action of insulin is desired
    4. The complex prevents the development of antibodies to exogenously administered insulin

<u>ONE BEST ANSWER</u>

12. _______   The drug of choice for the treatment of adrenogenital syndrome of the
               11β – hydroxylase deficiency type is:

               1. Progesterone
               2. Metyrapone
               3. Mitotane
               4. Hydrocortisone
               5. Estrogen

13. _______   The prolonged administration of prednisolone may produce all of the
               following side effects EXCEPT:

               1. Psychosis
               2. Peptic ulcer
               3. Hypertrophy of the adrenal cortex
               4. Osteoporosis
               5. Lymphopenia

14. _______   Which one of the following is the drug of choice for
               mineralocorticoid replacement therapy in patients with Addison's
               disease?

               1. Prednisone
               2. Cortisol
               3. Dexamethasone
               4. Aldosterone
               5. Fludrocortisone

15. _______   Epinephrine promotes glycogenolysis. The first enzyme to be
               stimulated by epinephrine in this process is:

               1. Protein kinase
               2. Glycogen synthase
               3. Phosphodiesterase
               4. Adenylate cyclase
               5. Phosphorylase

16. _______   Which of the following has been associated with the use of androgenic
               steroids?

               1. Increase in nitrogen retention and muscle mass
               2. Stimulation of growth of a latent prostatic carcinoma
               3. Increased sodium retention and formation of edema fluid
               4. Cholestatic jaundice (17-alkyl derivatives)
               5. All of the above

<u>ONE BEST ANSWER</u>

17. _______ The principle advantage of the use of dexamethasone over the use of hydrocortisone in the treatment of rheumatoid arthritis is?

    1. Less suppression of lymphatic tissue for the same anti-inflammatory response
    2. Less suppression of ACTH secretion for the same anti-inflammatory response
    3. Less liability for the induction of diabetes mellitus for the same anti-inflammatory response
    4. Less sodium retention for the same anti-inflammatory response

18. _______ Radioactive iodine in treatment of hyperthyroidism:

    1. High incidence of hypothyroidism
    2. Rapidly and efficiently trapped by the thyroid
    3. Indicated in older patients with heart disease
    4. Contraindicated during pregnancy
    5. All of the above

19. _______ Liotrix:

    1. Three to four times as potent as sodium levothyroxine
    2. Combination of synthetic T_4 and T_3 in a ratio of 4:1
    3. Dessicated thyroid powder standardized by bioassay
    4. Dessicated thyroid powder standardized on the basis of iodine content
    5. None of the above

20. _______ Levothyroxine toxicity:

    1. Agranulocytosis
    2. Lowered plasma cholesterol concentrations
    3. Depression
    4. Cardiac symptoms
    5. Aplastic anemia

<u>MATCHING</u>

The administration of cortisol, dexamethasone, ACTH, mitotane
(o,p-DDD) or metyrapone causes changes in plasma levels of ACTH,
desoxycortisol, cortisol and dehydroepiandrosterone (DEA), and
changes in urinary excretion of 17-hydroxycorticosteroids (17-OH-CS)
and 17-keto-steroids (17-KS). Match the changes in the laboratory
findings most likely to be observed in patients who received each of
the following agents.

	ACTH	Desoxy-cortisol	Cortisol	DEA	17-OH-CS	17-KS
1	↑	↑	↑	↑	↑	↑
2	↑	↓	↓	↓	↓	↓
3	↓	↓	↑	↓	↑	↓
4	↑	↑	↓	↑	↑	↑
5	↓	↓	↓	↓	↓	↓

21. _______ Cortisol

22. _______ Dexamethasone

23. _______ ACTH

24. _______ Mitotane

25. _______ Metyrapone

****

Match the following drugs with the most appropriate statement.

1. Norethindrone
2. Danazol
3. Mestranol
4. Estrogen
5. Progesterone

26. _______ Growth hormone of reproductive tissues in female; causes suppression
of FSH secretion

27. _______ Synthetic progestin; may be used alone as contraceptive agent in the
minidose pill

28. _______ Hormone that promotes relaxation of uterus; stimulates secretory
phase of cycle

29. _______ An "impeded" androgen, used for endometriosis

30. _______ Synthetic estrogen employed in a number of oral contraceptive
preparations

<u>MATCHING</u>

Match the terms listed in questions 31 - 33 with the appropriate description or explanation given below. Match the ONE best answer to each statement.

1. Thyroxine
2. Propylthiouracil
3. Both
4. Neither

31. _______ Diminishes secretion of endogenous thyroid hormone and inhibits uptake of iodide by the thyroid gland by a direct action on the secretion of TSH by the anterior pituitary

32. _______ Diminishes secretion of endogenous thyroid hormone by a mechanism which does not lower iodide uptake by the thyroid gland

33. _______ Used effectively in the treatment of hypothyroid states but its concentration cannot be estimated by determining protein bound iodine because it is not bound to plasma protein

<u>MULTIPLE TRUE-FALSE</u>
Directions: For each of the statements below, <u>ONE</u> or <u>MORE</u> of the completions given is correct.

1 - If only 1, 2 and 3 are correct
2 - If only 1 and 3 are correct
3 - If only 2 and 4 are correct
4 - If only 4 is correct
5 - If all are correct

34. _______ The administration of fluoxymesterone is contraindicated in patients who:

1. Are pregnant
2. Have carcinoma of the breast
3. Suffer from some liver dysfunction
4. Are cachectic

35. _______ Which of the following are true of the treatment of diabetic patients with sulfonylurea antidiabetic drugs?

1. Induces weight loss due to a central anorexic effect
2. Alleviates the progressive arteriosclerosis associated with diabetes
3. Decreases the incidence of bacterial infections because of their structural similarities to antibacterial sulfonamides
4. Ineffective in the absence of pancreatic insulin reserves

<u>MULTIPLE TRUE-FALSE</u>
<u>Directions Summarized:</u>

1	2	3	4	5
1,2,3	1,3	2,4	4	all are
only	only	only	only	correct

36. _______ The steroid hormone 1,25-dihydroxycholecalciferol:

1. Is secreted by the kidneys
2. Is derived from Vitamin D
3. Stimulates intestinal calcium transport
4. Stimulates calcium reabsorption from the bone matrix

37. _______ Testosterone can cause which of the following?

1. Masculinization
2. Acne
3. Feminization
4. Jaundice

38. _______ Testosterone cannot be administered orally because:

1. It is a gastric irritant
2. It is not absorbed
3. It is excreted unaltered
4. It is rapidly metabolized by the liver

39. _______ Which of the following is the most life-threatening result of adrenal insufficiency?

1. Decreased gluconeogenesis
2. Lymphoid hyperplasia
3. The inability to excrete a water load
4. Loss of sodium ion in the urine

40. _______ Vasopressin:

1. Is a long-chained polypeptide of unknown composition
2. Is useful in the treatment of shock
3. Has its primary action in the treatment of edema by promoting water loss
4. Is produced in the hypothalamus and stored in the posterior pituitary

41. _______ Oxytocin administration:

1. Induces vigorous contractions in the non-pregnant uterus which is in the secretory phase of the menstrual cycle
2. Promotes milk ejection in nursing mothers
3. Can induce abortion early in pregnancy
4. Increases the frequency of contractions of the uterus late in pregnancy

<u>MULTIPLE TRUE-FALSE</u>
Directions Summarized:

1	2	3	4	5
1,2,3	1,3	2,4	4	all are
only	only	only	only	correct

42. _______ Small doses of progestin (e.g. "minipill") are contraceptive because
they:

1. Alter the structure of the endometrium
2. Inhibit ovulation
3. Change the consistency of the cervical mucus
4. Induce excessive vomiting

43. _______ Clomiphene:

1. Inhibits FSH and LH secretion
2. Increases the incidence of multiple births
3. Is a potent contraceptive agent
4. Is an ovulatory agent

44. _______ Estrogen therapy may be indicated for:

1. Failure of ovarian development
2. Painful menstruation
3. Atrophic vaginitis
4. Prevention of heart attacks

45. _______ Which of the following could result in an alteration of the daily
insulin dosage for a diabetic patient?

1. Prolonged exercise
2. Pregnancy
3. Marked weight loss
4. Surgery

ANSWERS

1.	4	
2.	3	
3.	3	Insulin acts to decrease gluconeogenesis as part of its hypoglycemic action
4.	4	
5.	1	2 is a correct statement but not the mechanism of action.
6.	4	
7.	3	One or two large doses have no adverse effects. Treatment of the other conditions require chronic dosing schedules.
8.	5	
9.	3	
10.	3	If anything, 2,3 diphosphoglycerate would be decreased due to phosphate loss secondary to diuresis.
11.	3	Protamine insulin is insoluble and has all the actions of regular insulin.
12.	4	This is a virilizing, hypertensive syndrome. The treatment is hydrocortisone (cortisol) to shut off ACTH thus decreasing the production of androgens and sodium retaining hormones.
13.	3	It would produce atrophy by decreasing ACTH production.
14.	5	This compound is orally effective and has marked salt retaining activity.
15.	4	
16.	5	
17.	4	All of the others are directly related to the activity of the agent as an anti-inflammatory agent.
18.	5	
19.	2	
20.	4	
21.	3	
22.	5	Both cortisol and dexamethasone would decrease ACTH but only cortisol would increase cortisol and 17-OH-KS.
23.	1	ACTH would increase ACTH and cortisol.
24.	2	Mitotane would increase ACTH because of loss of inhibition by cortisol. Synthesis of all steroids decreased.
25.	4	Metyrapone inhibits 11- -hydroxylase; therefore, cortisol but not DOC would decrease and ACTH would increase.
26.	4	
27.	1	
28.	5	
29.	2	
30.	3	
31.	1	
32.	2	
33.	4	
34.	2	
35.	4	
36.	5	
37.	1	
38.	4	
39.	4	
40.	4	

41.	3	Oxytocin is relatively ineffective early in pregnancy or on the non-pregnant uterus; however, vasopressin is active.
42.	2	
43.	3	
44.	1	
45.	5	

SECTION VII: <u>CHEMOTHERAPY</u>

CHEMOTHERAPY OF MICROBIAL DISEASES

I. ANTISEPTICS AND GERMICIDES

A. DETERGENTS:

1. <u>Anionic</u>: (ordinary soaps, sodium alkyl sulfonates, etc.) effective
against some Gram positive organisms; maximum effect at low pH;
usually a Na^+ or K^+ salt of long chain fatty acid; salt dissociates
to give a polar and non-polar end; use alcohol to remove.

2. <u>Cationic</u>: (tetra-substituted ammonium chloride; benzalkonium
chloride is an example;) effective against Gram positive and Gram
negative organisms; maximum effect at high pH; slow acting; can
protect organisms under surface film; anionic detergents neutralize
cationic detergents; inactive against spores; well tolerated.

3. <u>Nonionic</u>: Are not antimicrobial.

B. PHENOLS (Probably also act as detergents):

1. <u>Phenol</u>: irritant; not too effective; used as standard to measure
the effectiveness of other antimicrobials as disinfectants (the
phenol coefficient); classic substance, but too weak and toxic.

2. <u>Cresol</u>: 3x as potent as phenol; no more toxic; cheap; found in
Lysol brand disinfectants.

3. <u>Hexylresorcinol</u>: 50x as potent as phenol; activity also as a
broad-spectrum antihelminthic

4. <u>Hexachlorophene</u>: can be incorporated into soaps and detergents;
when used over a long period of time, forms a persistent monolayer
on the skin which exerts a prolonged antibacterial action against
Gram positive microbes; monolayer removed by other detergents;
useful for elective surgery (plastic); potential CNS toxicity in
pediatric uses.

C. ALCOHOLS:

Generally effective. Activity increases and solubility decreases
with chain length.

1. <u>Ethanol</u>: Rapid acting; limited effectiveness against Gram positive
and Gram negative organisms at concentrations between 50-95%; also
exerts cleansing action; a taxable beverage; miscible with water.

2. <u>Isopropyl alcohol</u>: Lower vapor pressure than ethyl alcohol;
doesn't evaporate as rapidly; causes less rusting of surgical
instruments than does ethanol; not a beverage; cheaper than
ethanol; miscible with water.

D. HALOGENS:

1. <u>Chlorine</u>: Undissociated hypochlorous acid is effective; dissolves blood clots; effectiveness depends upon pH, and the amount of nonspecific protein which is present. Supplied as sodium hypochlorite.

2. <u>Chloramines</u>: less irritating to tissues than hypochlorite; do not dissolve blood clots; depot preparation of chlorine dissociates in H_2O to hypochlorous acid.

3. <u>Iodine</u>: broad spectrum antibacterial action, can be locally irritating. Supplied as tincture or solution; IODOPHORS (providone iodine) are less irritating: kills fungi.

E. METALS:

1. <u>Mercury</u>: ($HgCl_2$, thimerosal) bacteriostatic over a wide range of concentrations; action reversed by sulfhydryl compounds; inorganic salts more toxic than organic mercurial compounds.

2. <u>Silver</u>: Can be caustic, astringent or antiseptic, depending upon the concentration of Ag ions; silver nitrate has high degree of ionization and is precipitated by chloride ions in tissues; silver proteinates have very low concentration of silver ions and do not precipitate with tissue chloride ion; rarely used today; with chronic use accumulate photochemical silver products in the skin, which imparts blue color to skin (argyria).

F. OXIDANTS (not an important group of agents today) increase oxygen tension:

1. <u>Peroxides (hydrogen, sodium, zinc)</u>: Release oxygen; foam and bubble; cleanse and debride.

2. <u>Permanganate</u>: Forms highly insoluble manganese dioxide; stains sheets brown.

3. <u>Perborate</u>: Still used by dentists as mouth wash.

II. URINARY ANTISEPTICS

Substances which can be given by mouth, are distributed throughout the body fluids (but do not exert a significant anti-bacterial action in these fluids), and are excreted in the urine (where they DO exert antibacterial effects).

A. METHENAMINE:

Dissociates into formaldehyde (the active material) and ammonia in acid urine.

B. MANDELIC ACID:

Acidifies the urine, is antibacterial in its own right and can be added to methenamine; mixture known as mandelamine.

C. NITROFURANTOIN:

Bacteriostatic activity against a number of urinary tract pathogens, by an unknown mechanism. Resistance rarely develops. Hypersensitivity reactions, nausea and vomiting are limitations to its usefulness; peripheral neuropathy occasionally seen; a crystalline form of nitrofurantoin has a reduced incidence of gastrointestinal intolerance.

D. NALIDIXIC ACID:

Nausea, vomiting, skin rashes, and CNS effects are common; microbial resistance develops very rapidly; inhibits bacterial DNA synthesis.

E. TRIMETHOPRIM:

Selective inhibition of bacterial dihydrofolate reductase. May be bacteriostatic or bactericidal. Only approved indication is for uncomplicated urinary tract infections caused by susceptible organisms.

III. SULFONAMIDES (Sulfas)---derivatives of p-aminobenzenesulfonamide

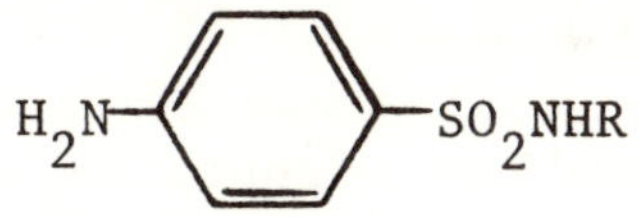

$$H_2N-\!\!\bigcirc\!\!-SO_2NHR$$

A. MECHANISM OF ANTIBACTERIAL ACTION:

Structurally similar to p-aminobenzoic acid (PABA), and block folic acid synthesis in microbes which must synthesize folic acid from PABA.
Bacteriostatic; not bactericidal in the concentrations which can be achieved in most body tissues and fluids (exception: the high concentrations which are achieved in urine can be bactericidal).

B. SPECTRUM:

Broad spectrum, effective against most gram positive bacteria, many gram negative bacteria, nocardia, actinomyces, chlamydia and plasmodia.

C. ABSORPTION, DISTRIBUTION AND EXCRETION:

Readily absorbed after oral administration. Sodium salts may be given i.v., but are strongly alkaline and cause pain and tissue sloughing if extravasated.
Sulfonamides are 20-90% bound to plasma albumin, depending on the sulfonamide and its concentration. Free (unbound) drug is distributed to total body water.

Approximately 20% of a sulfonamide dose is oxidized; other metabolic products are acetylated and glucuronide conjugates.

Sulfonamides are eliminated in urine by glomerular filtration and tubular secretion.

D. TOXICITY:

Renal crystallization caused by precipitation of insoluble sulfonamides in acid urine; drug allergy; may cause toxicity to the hematopoietic system (acute hemolytic anemia, thrombocytopenia, etc.).

C. INDIVIDUAL AGENTS: Do not differ in antimicrobial activity

1. <u>Short-acting sulfonamides</u>

Rapidly absorbed and excreted into urine, giving high urinary concentrations. Usually given 4 times daily.

   a. Sulfacytine
   b. Sulfadiazine
   c. Sulfamethizole
   d. Sulfisoxazole

2. <u>Intermediate-acting sulfonamide</u>

Sulfamethoxazole; longer half-life allows dosing at 8 to 12 hour intervals.

3. <u>Sulfonamide combinations</u>

   a. Trisulfapyrimidines - contains equal amounts of sulfadiazine, sulfamerazine and sulfamethazine. An old "triple sulfa" formulation for additive antibacterial effects but less chance of crystalluria.
   b. Sulfathiazole, sulfacetamide and sulfabenzamide - vaginal cream of questionable efficacy
   c. Sulfamethoxazole and trimethoprim - synergistic activity of a sulfonamide plus dihydrofolate reductase inhibitor.

4. <u>Miscellaneous Sulfonamides and related compounds</u>

   a. Sulfacetamide - an acetylated derivative; the soluble sodium salt is widely used for ophthalmic infections.
   b. Sulfapyridine - obsolete due to high risk of crystalluria, except as an alternative to dapsone for dermatitis herpetiformis.
   c. Sulfasalazine - often effective in treating acute exacerbations of ulcerative colitis; however, this action appears to be unrelated to antibacterial action.
   d. Mafenide - not a true sulfonamide; used for burns.
   e. Silver sulfadiazine - less painful than mafenide and does not cause metabolic acidosis.

D. MAJOR USES:

Urinary tract infections; with streptomycin in plague, tularemia, possibly <u>H</u>. <u>influenzae</u> meningitis; nocardia; actinomycosis; resistant <u>falciparum</u> malaria.

IV. BETA-LACTAM ANTIBIOTICS

Beta-lactam antibiotics have been widely investigated for use in medicine because of their high degree of selective toxicity against bacteria. Individual beta-lactam antibiotics may differ widely in their antibacterial spectra, pharmacokinetic properties, and resistance to hydrolysis by beta-lactamases.

A. MECHANISM OF ACTION: All beta-lactam antibiotics bind covalently to penicillin binding proteins (PBP's) of bacterial cell membranes. Various strains of bacteria may have differing numbers of PBPs, but all appear to be involved in some stage of bacterial cell wall synthesis. Incubation of susceptible bacteria with beta-lactam antibiotics may result in morphological abnormalities and cell death. Cell lysis, when it occurs, may result from uncontrolled action of bacterial lytic enzymes. Beta-lactam antibiotics may be bacteriostatic to some strains of bacteria at low drug concentrations. Because of the selective action of beta-lactam antibiotics against cell wall synthesis, these drugs are most effective against actively growing bacterial cultures.

B. METABOLISM AND EXCRETION: Most beta-lactam antibiotics are excreted unchanged in the urine. Both glomerular filtration and tubular secretion contribute to the urinary secretion of beta-lactam antibiotics; probenecid will inhibit tubular secretion. A few agents are excreted primarily into the bile.

C. TOXICITY: Allergic reactions are the most common toxic complications, and there is a small incidence (5-10%) of cross-reactivity among the penicillins and cephalosporins. Some agents have unique toxicities of low incidence which are not characteristic of most beta-lactam antibiotics. CNS dysfunction (lethargy, confusion, seizures) may occur with high blood and CSF levels.

D. PENICILLINS:

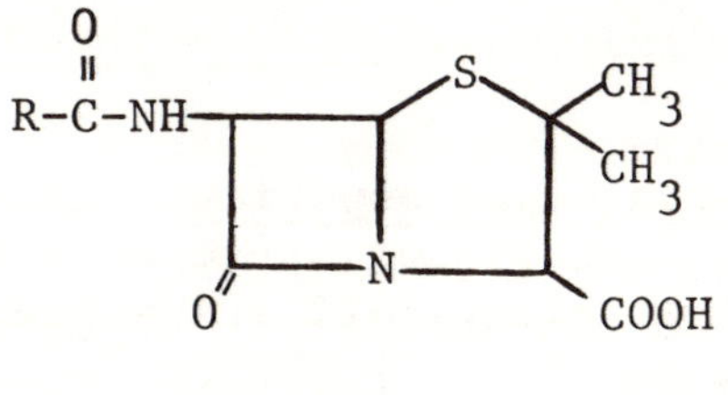

$$\text{R-C-NH} \quad \overset{\text{O}}{\underset{\text{O}}{\|}} \quad \text{S} \quad \text{CH}_3 \quad \text{CH}_3 \quad \text{N} \quad \text{COOH}$$

1. <u>Narrow spectrum: Gram positive</u>

a. Penicillin G (Benzyl penicillin) - The prototypic penicillin; should be given parenterally since oral absorption is erratic due to instability in gastric acid.
b. Penicillin V (Phenoxymethyl penicillin) - Acid stable, for oral use only.
c. Penicillinase-Resistant penicillins

Parenteral: Methicillin (prototype); oxacillin; nafcillin
Oral: Oxacillin; cloxacillin; dicloxacillin; nafcillin

2. <u>Narrow spectrum: Gram negative</u>

   a. Amdinocillin - Binds to a unique PBP. Has weak antibacterial activity alone, but is synergistic with other beta-lactam antibiotics which also are active against gram-negative bacteria.

3. <u>"Extended Spectrum" Penicillins</u>: possess activity against some important gram positive and gram-negative pathogens

   a. <u>Amino penicillins</u>: Ampicillin (prototype). Amoxicillin has superior absorption. Other aminopenicillins include: Hetacillin, Cyclacillin and Bacampicillin.

   b. "Anti-pseudomonal" penicillins: Ticarcillin and Carbenicillin.

4. <u>Broad Spectrum Penicillins</u> - Improved activity against gram-negative pathogens, including <u>Pseudomonas</u> <u>aeruginosa</u>. Piperacillin, mezlocillin, and azlocillin.

E. CEPHALOSPORINS: Includes the true cephalosporins (produced from <u>Cephalosporium</u> spp.) and cephamycins (produced from Streptomyces spp.). Cephamycins possess a 7-methoxy substitution on the beta-lactam ring which results in greater resistance to beta-lactamases. The possibility of chemical substitutions on both sides of the ring structure (R_1 and R_2) results in a number of agents with differing spectra and pharmacokinetic properties. Cephalosporins are classified into "generations" on the basis of their antibacterial spectrum.

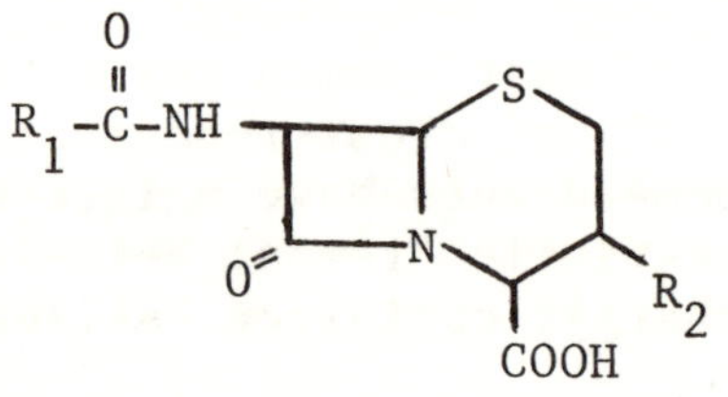

Cephalosporins

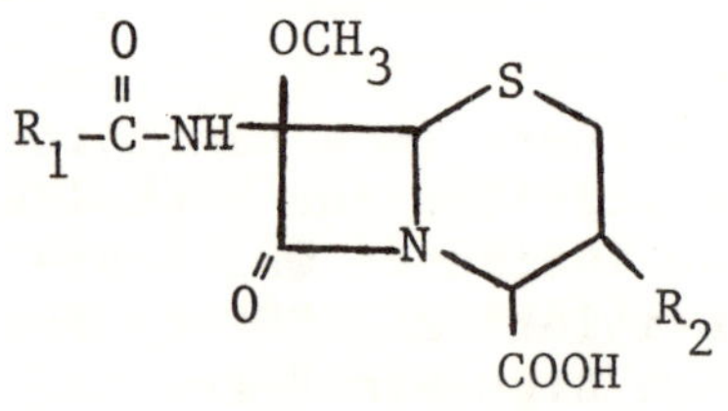

Cephamycins

1. <u>First-Generation Cephalosporins</u> - Most important for gram-positive activity. Essentially no difference among various drugs in antibacterial effects. All are susceptible to beta-lactamase inactivation.

   a. <u>Parenteral agents</u>: Cefazolin, Cephalothin, Cephapirin, Cephradine

   b. <u>Oral agents</u>: Cephalexin, Cefadroxil, Cephradine

   c. <u>Summary</u>: There are few important differences among the first generation cephalosporins. <u>Cefazolin</u> has the longest half-life and is least irritating of the parenteral agents, so is the best choice for i.m. injection. The absorption of <u>cefadroxil</u> after oral administration is somewhat greater than the other oral agents.

2. <u>Second-Generation Cephalosporins</u> - In general, have activity against a greater number of gram-negative pathogens than first generation agents, especially <u>Hemophilus influenzae</u>. However, first-generation agents are preferred for most gram-positive indications, and third-generation agents are usually more active against gram-negative pathogens.

    a. <u>Parenteral agents</u>: Cefamandole, Cefuroxime, Cefonicid, Ceforanide, Cefoxitin.

    b. <u>Oral agent</u>: Cefachlor

    c. <u>Summary</u>: Cefoxitin (a cephamycin) is the only notable drug of this class because of its good anaerobic activity. Some individual features of other agents may make them useful in selected patients: long half-life (cefonicid); penetration into CSF (cefuroxime); absence of sodium in formulation (ceforanide).

3. <u>Third Generation Cephalosporins</u> - Broad spectrum antimicrobial drugs; however, potency against gram-positive microbes is generally inferior to first-generation agents. All third generation cephalosporins are resistant to hydrolysis by beta-lactamases. None are orally effective.

Cefotaxime	Ceftriaxone
Moxalactam	Ceftazidime
Cefoperazone	Cefotetan
Ceftizoxime	

Individual third generation cephalosporins have properties which may offer particular clinical advantages or unexpected toxicity. These properties are not necessarily shared by all third-generation cephalosporins.

    a. <u>Advantageous properties</u>

       i. Penetration into CSF (Ceftazidime, Moxalactam)
      ii. Biliary excretion (Cefoperazone, Ceftriaxone)
    iii. Long half-life (Ceftriaxone)
     iv. Anti-pseudomonal activity (Ceftazidime)
      v. Anaerobic activity (Cefotetan - a cephamycin, and Moxalactam)

    b. <u>Unusual toxicities</u>

       i. Disulfiram-like effects (Moxalactam, Cefoperazone)
      ii. Hypoprothrombinemia (A potential problem with all broad spectrum antibiotics, possibly due to diminished synthesis of vitamin K by intestinal microbes, but seems particularly problematic with moxalactam).

F. OXAPENEMS:

Clavulanic Acid

Clavulanic acid is the only marketed oxapenem. It has poor
antimicrobial potency, but is an irreversible inhibitor of
beta-lactamase. Clavulanic acid is combined with other beta-lactam
antibiotics to increase their effectiveness.

G. CARBAPENEMS:

Imipenem

   Imipenem was introduced in 1985 as the first "thienamycin"
antibiotic to be marketed. Imipenem binds to all PBPs and has the
broadest spectrum of any beta-lactam antibiotic. It is also an
irreversible beta-lactamase inhibitor.
   Imipenem is metabolized by a renal peptidase, and little active
drug could be recovered in urine. To circumvent this metabolism, a
specific inhibitor of the renal enzyme, cilistatin, was
synthesized. Cilistatin also prevents renal toxicity sometimes
observed with imipenem alone.
   A 1:1 combination of imipenem:cilistatin is available.

H. MONOBACTAMS: Monobactams are unusual beta-lactam antibiotics in
    that the beta-lactam ring is not fused with another ring. A number
    of monobactam antibiotics have been discovered, and are under
    study.

1. Aztreonam: Aztreonam is a potent, narrow-spectrum antibiotic,
    with activity only against gram-negative bacteria. It is
    highly stable to beta-lactamases, does not induce
    beta-lactamase enzymes, and shows poor immune cross-reactivity
    with other beta-lactam antibiotics. Aztreonam is synergistic
    with other beta-lactam antibiotics and the aminoglycosides.

V. AMINOGLYCOSIDES

A. MECHANISM OF ACTION: All aminoglycosides inhibit bacterial protein synthesis. Streptomycin binds to a specific site on the 30S ribosomal subunit, but other aminoglycosides bind to sites on both the 30S and 50S ribosomal subunits. The antibacterial action may be related to inhibition of protein synthesis, or to disruption of cell membrane function caused by the transport of the ionized antibiotics into the bacterial cells.

B. SPECTRUM: Usually bactericidal for many gram positive and gram negative bacteria. Because aminoglycosides are actively transported into a bacterial cell by an oxygen-dependent enzyme system, only aerobic bacteria are sensitive to these drugs.

C. ABSORPTION, DISTRIBUTION AND EXCRETION: Not absorbed from the GI tract; readily absorbed from intramuscular or subcutaneous sites. Distributed to extracellular water; poor penetration to CSF (even when meninges are inflammed). Excreted in urine after glomerular filtration of parent compound.

D. TOXICITY: Aminoglycosides cause renal toxicity, and may damage both vestibular and auditory functions of the eighth cranial nerve. Allergic reactions occasionally occur.

E. INDIVIDUAL AGENTS AND USES:

1. Streptomycin – Use generally restricted to tuberculosis, bacterial endocarditis, plague, and tularemia.
2. Neomycin – Most toxic and used only topically, or orally for gut sterilization.
3. Kanamycin – Older agent, seldom used.
4. Gentamicin ⎤   Essentially comparable agents for systemic use in
5. Tobramycin ⎟—   serious infections. May be slight differences in
6. Netilmicin ⎦   bacterial sensitivity or potential for
                     renal/auditory toxicity.
7. Amikacin – A derivative of Kanamycin which resists inactivation by many bacterial enzymes; should be reserved for susceptible infections resistant to other aminoglycosides.

VI. TETRACYCLINES

A. MECHANISM OF ACTION: Preferentially bound to 30S subunit of microbial ribosome. Seems to interfere with binding of amino acyl-t-RNA and inhibit chain termination. Drugs are bacteriostatic, not bactericidal.

B. SPECTRUM: Broad spectrum agents, effective against gram positive and gram negative bacteria, rickettsia, chlamydia, spirochetes, amebiasis.

C. ABSORPTION, DISTRIBUTION AND EXCRETION: Incompletely absorbed after oral administration, and absorption is further delayed by food, calcium salts, and aluminum salts. (Exception: The oral absorption of doxycycline is superior to the other tetracyclines, and is virtually unaffected by food.) Tetracyclines are distributed in total body water.

Chlortetracycline and demeclocycline are extensively metabolized by
the body; other tetracyclines to a lesser extent (so that renal
excretion is relatively more important in determining blood levels).
Kidney elimination is least important with doxycycline.

D. TOXICITY: GI disturbances; superinfection; damage to forming teeth and
bones; liver damage, particularly in pregnant women who get the drug
intravenously; photosensitization (particularly with demeclocycline).
Parenteral forms are irritating.

E. USES: Rickettsial infections; chlamydial infections; sexually
transmitted diseases; brucellosis. Often used as alternate therapy in
penicillin-allergic patients.

F. INDIVIDUAL AGENTS: The individual tetracyclines differ from one
another only in the duration of their action and the stability of the
drugs in the body. All are broad spectrum antibiotics.

1. <u>Rapidly eliminated</u>: Tetracycline-(Prototype drug of this group);
Chlortetracycline; Oxytetracycline.

2. <u>More slowly eliminated</u>: Demeclocycline and Methacycline.

3. <u>Long-acting</u>: Doxycycline and Minocycline.

VII. CHLORAMPHENICOL

A. MECHANISM OF ACTION: Attaches at P sites of 50S subunit of microbial
ribosome. Inhibits functional attachment to amino acyl end of AA-t-RNA
to 50S subunit, inhibiting transpeptidation. The drug is
bacteriostatic, not bactericidal.

B. SPECTRUM: Broad spectrum antibiotic, more effective than tetracyclines
against typhoid fever and other <u>Salmonella</u> infections. Good activity
against many anaerobic bacteria and rickettsia.

C. ABSORPTION, DISTRIBUTION AND EXCRETION: Chloramphenicol is well
absorbed after oral administration, and is distributed into total body
water. A special feature is excellent penetration into CSF, ocular
fluids and joint fluids. Chloramphenicol is rapidly excreted in urine,
10% as chloramphenicol, 90% as glucuronide.

D. TOXICITY: BLOOD DYSCRASIAS: Irreversible aplastic anemia is most
serious effect. Reversible bone marrow depression may also occur.
Gray baby syndrome in neonates due to deficient glucuronidation of
drug. Superinfections.

E. USES: Broad spectrum and penetration into CSF make it useful in
meningitis; rickettsial infections; anaerobic infections; Salmonella
infections. The risk of aplastic anemia limits its application to
situations where safer drugs are not likely to be effective.

VIII. ERYTHROMYCIN (a macrolide antibiotic)

A. MECHANISM OF ACTION: Binds to P site of 50S ribosomal subunit. Blocks protein synthesis when a large amino acid or a polypeptide is in the P site.

B. SPECTRUM: Narrow, gram-positive spectrum, similar to penicillin G. Resistance develops rapidly.

C. ABSORPTION, DISTRIBUTION AND EXCRETION: Oral absorption is adequate with free base or stearate salts; better absorption (higher blood levels) with estolate salt. Erythromycin is distributed into total body water, but penetration to CSF is poor, even when meninges are inflammed. The drug is extensively destroyed by the body, so that the renal function of the patient is unimportant for the dose.

D. TOXICITY: Usually well tolerated; reversible intrahepatic obstructive jaundice seen most commonly with estolate salt.

E. USES: Often used as a substitute for penicillin V in allergic patients. Erythromycin is the drug of choice for Legionnaires disease, and is useful in diphtheria, pertussis and chlamydial infections.

IX. LINCOMYCIN AND CLINDAMYCIN (7-chlorolincomycin)

A. MECHANISM OF ACTION: Attach to 50S ribosomal subunit, at or near the erythromycin attachment site. Chemically unlike, but pharmacologically similar to, erythromycin.

B. SPECTRUM: Narrow gram-positive spectrum, but with excellent activity against anaerobic bacteria. Clindamycin is more potent antimicrobial agent than Lincomycin.

C. ABSORPTION, DISTRIBUTION AND EXCRETION: Lincomycin is poorly absorbed after oral administration, and is seldom used clinically. The oral absorption of clindamycin is excellent, and is not affected by food. These drugs are widely distributed in the body (but reach only low concentrations in CSF, even when meninges are inflammed) and penetrate well into bone. Both drugs are metabolized extensively, and excreted primarily in bile and feces.

D. TOXICITY: Diarrhea is most common adverse effect. Antibiotic-associated colitis is most common with clindamycin. Skin rashes and reversible changes in hepatic enzymes in serum may also occur.

E. USES: Clindamycin is useful for therapy of anaerobic infections, including <u>Bacteroides</u> <u>fragilis</u>. It is potentially useful as a penicillin substitute, but is more toxic than erythromycin.

X. VANCOMYCIN

Inhibits bacterial cell wall synthesis at a different step than the beta-lactam antibiotics. Usually bactericidal. Not absorbed orally; when given i.v., causes thrombophlebitis. Ototoxic and nephrotoxic. An

alternative to penicillin in life-threatening infections in
penicillin-allergic patients or penicillin-resistant staphylococcus.

XI. MISCELLANEOUS ANTIBACTERIAL DRUGS

A. SPECTINOMYCIN:

Spectinomycin is chemically related to the aminoglycosides. It
binds at the 30S subunit of the microbial ribosome, but at a site
different from that of streptomycin. Drug seems to be bacteriostatic
rather than bactericidal, because of reversible bond. Not absorbed
orally; given intramuscularly. Used exclusively for the one-shot
treatment of gonorrhea; ineffective against syphilis.

B. POLYMYXIN B AND COLISTIN

Polypeptide antibiotics; effective primarily against Gram negative
organisms, particularly; Pseudomonas; reversible renal damage and
various neurological changes limit the usefulness of these drugs to
topical applications; they may be used systemically in life-threatening
infections resistant to safer antibiotics; not absorbed orally; usually
given i.v.

C. BACITRACIN:

A polypeptide antibiotic, acts on bacterial cell walls; effective
against Gram positive organisms; renal toxicity limits usefulness of
Bacitracin to topical use, but it may be useful in life-threatening
infections resistant to safer antibiotics; not absorbed orally; given
i.m.

D. METRONIDAZOLE:

A nitroimidazole compound active against many anaerobic bacteria
and protozoa; well absorbed after oral administration; may cause
various neurological effects and sodium retention; various G.I.
symptoms.

E. ANTI-TUBERCULOSIS DRUGS:

1. AMINOSALICYLIC ACID (PAS):

Tuberculostatic; resistance develops more slowly than to other
anti-TB drugs; readily absorbed from the GI tract, does not enter
the CSF; acetylated in the liver, rapidly excreted by the kidneys
(probenecid slows renal tubular secretion); side effects include
gastric irritation, allergic reactions, hematological disorders;
given with other antitubercular drugs, chiefly to delay the
emergence of microbial resistance.

2. ISONIAZID (INH)

Tuberculostatic or tuberculocidal, depending upon
concentration; resistance develops rapidly; readily absorbed
orally, widely distributed through body, enters CSF and caseous

masses; causes pyridoxal deficiency (peripheral neuritis in adults, convulsions in children); administration of vitamin B_6 prevents these signs; INH reacts chemically with pyridoxal; there are genetic differences in the rate at which individuals acetylate (and inactivate) isoniazid; well tolerated, widely used.

3. ETHAMBUTOL

Orally absorbed, with fewer GI side-effects than aminosalicylic acid; probably an RNA-synthesis inhibitor; resistance develops slowly; usually well tolerated; retrobulbar neuritis (visual field defects) seen occasionally at high doses; may replace aminosalicylic acid in treatment schedules.

4. RIFAMPIN (one of a family of rifamycins)

Orally effective against TB and other microbes; seems to inhibit DNA-directed RNA synthesis; resistance develops readily; well-tolerated, expensive, but very promising; well-distributed, gets into CNS.

F. ANTI-LEPROSY DRUGS

1. DAPSONE (DDS)

Antagonized by PABA; long half-life permits once-a-week administration; hemolysis is most common side effect; exacerbation of lepromatous leprosy may occur.

2. THALIDOMIDE

Effective against erythema nodosum leprosum.

XII. ANTIFUNGAL AGENTS

A. NYSTATIN:

Not absorbed orally, too irritating to be used parenterally; only used for cutaneous or mucocutaneous Candida infections.

B. AMPHOTERICIN B:

Not absorbed orally; given by intravenous infusion. It has a broad antifungal spectrum, and is effective against most systemic mycotic infections. In spite of severe toxicity (including renal damage), amphotericin B is the drug of choice for most systemic fungal infections. Acts on fungal cell membrane.

C. GRISEOFULVIN:

Given orally for the treatment of persistent ring-worm infections. Prolonged (expensive) administration required. A variety of side effects have been reported (GI disturbances, skin rashes, CNS signs).

D. FLUCYTOSINE:

Effective orally for systemic infections of Candida or
Cryptococcus. Use with extreme caution in patients with impaired renal
function. Close monitoring of hematologic, renal and hepatic status is
essential.

E. MICONAZOLE AND KETOCONAZOLE:

Miconazole is given by i.v. infusion and ketoconazole is given
orally for a variety of severe systemic fungal infections. Rashes and
GI symptoms are common. Ketoconazole may cause serious hepatotoxicity.

XIII. ANTIVIRAL DRUGS

A. AMANTADINE:

Water-soluble hydrocarbon inhibits viral replication at an early
step, blocks uncoating; completely absorbed from GI tract, excreted
unchanged in urine, $t_{\frac{1}{2}}$ of 20 hr; CNS toxicity (nervousness, confusion,
insomnia, lightheadedness, hallucinations), usually transient;
prophylactic use against influenza A strains in high risk patients;
treatment of influenza A (reduces symptoms and duration of illness),
must be initiated within 24-48 hrs after onset of symptoms.

B. VIDARABINE:

An analog of adenosine (adenine arabinoside); must be
phosphorylated in cell; inhibits viral DNA polymerase; administered
i.v. in large volumes of fluid, rapidly deaminated in liver and plasma,
metabolites excreted in urine; toxicities: GI disturbances, skin rash,
neurologic abnormalities (rare); uses: herpes simplex encephalitis,
herpes simplex in neonates, herpes-zoster in suppressed patients,
herpes simplex keratitis (topically).

C. ACYCLOVIR:

An analogue of guanosine (acycloguanosine); selective toxicity
depends on virus-specified thymidine kinase, inhibits viral DNA
polymerase; poorly absorbed by oral route, excreted unchanged in urine,
$t_{\frac{1}{2}}$ = 2.5 h; minimal toxicity: renal toxicity when i.v.; headache,
nausea, rash when oral; genital herpes, herpes diseases in
immunocompromized patients.

D. IDOXURIDINE:

An analogue of thymidine; requires phosphorylation, incorporation
into DNA causes breakage, mutations, errors in transcription; systemic
toxicity: myelosuppression; topical toxicity: irritation, pain,
edema; limited use as an alternative topical treatment for herpes
simplex keratitis.

E. RIBAVIRIN:

A synthetic nucleoside (authentic ribose, fraudulent base with some similarity to guanine); effective against RSV and influenza viruses (A & B); mechanism unknown; administered by aerosol because of systemic toxicity (bone marrow depression); infants and children with severe, lower respiratory tract RSV.

F. INTERFERON:

Three types (alpha, beta and gamma); species specific; bind to receptors on surface membrane, multiple mechanisms produce the "antiviral state", immune effects are important; broad antiviral specificity; toxicities: extreme fatigue and numbness are dose-limiting; fever, mild leukopenia and thrombocytopemia; headache, myalgia.

CHEMOTHERAPY OF NEOPLASTIC DISEASES
(CANCER CHEMOTHERAPY)

A. GENERAL

A number of neoplastic diseases can be cured with drugs alone or with drugs in combination with other modalities (choriocarcinoma, Hodgkin's disease, acute leukemia, Burkitt's lymphoma, testicular carcinoma, Wilm's tumor, rhabdomyosarcoma, Ewing's sarcoma, retinoblastoma and diffuse histiocytic lymphoma). Adjuvant chemotherapy in combination with surgery and/or radiotherapy has increased survival rates for a number of solid tumors. However, the most prevalent forms of human cancer respond poorly or not at all to chemotherapy.

Cancer chemotherapeutic agents generally have low therapeutic indices and potentially lethal toxicities. In some cases the cancer patient may be best served by not being given drugs that cause serious toxic effects without prolonging life or improving its quality.

An understanding of cell kinetics is essential for the proper use of anticancer agents. Most anticancer drugs kill dividing cells (are proliferation dependent); thus, tumors with a high growth fraction are most susceptible (certain leukemias and lymphomas, small proliferating tumors, "recruited" tumor cells, micrometastases). The killing of tumor cells follows first order kinetics. To produce a cure, therapy must continue until the last tumor cell is gone. Agents which act preferentially on tumor cells in a given phase of the cell cycle are called cycle phase specific.

Many of the toxic effects of anticancer drugs are due to cytotoxic effects on normal tissues which have high proportions of dividing cells. These tissues include the bone marrow (cytopenias, increased risk of infection or activation of latent infection, immunosuppression, hemorrhage), digestive tract (oral and/or intestinal ulceration, diarrhea), hair root (alopecia), gonads (menstrual irregularities, amenorrhea, infertility, impaired spermatogenesis, sterility), repairing tissues (impaired healing) and fetus (teratogenesis). Anticancer drugs frequently produce nausea and vomitting which can be ameliorated with phenothiazines or cannabinoids. The release of nucleic acid breakdown products following a very large cell kill can result in hyperuricemia and renal damage; hyperuricemia is prevented with allopurinol. Many anticancer drugs are mutagenic and carcinogenic.

Cancer chemotherapy usually involves a combination of drugs. Ideally, drugs are selected which are effective when used alone, and have different mechanisms of action, minimally overlapping toxicities and no cross resistance. Doses close to the regular doses for each drug as a single agent can be used to optimize the cytotoxic effects without getting additive toxicity; the development of drug resistance is diminished.

B. ALKYLATING AGENTS

Bind covalently to DNA and other cell constituents, main effect is inhibition of DNA replication and transcription; proliferation dependent and cycle phase nonspecific. Repair of damage can occur; high rate of repair may be a cause of resistance. Alkylating agents generally are cross-resistant.

1. <u>Mechlorethamine</u>: the first anticancer drug to be widely used clinically; newer, better-tolerated drugs are more often used today; i.v., highly-reactive; potent vessicant; bone-marrow depression is dose-limiting

toxicity; severe nausea and vomiting; local reaction and phlebitis, alopecia, diarrhea, oral ulcers. Used mainly in MOPP regimen.

2. Cyclophosphamide: Most widely used alkylating agent; requires cytochrome P-450 mediated metabolism for activation; nonvessicant; oral or i.v.; bone marrow depression is dose-limiting; alopecia is prominent; immunosuppression is prominent; sterile hemorrhagic cystitis is common but preventable with adequate hydration; pulmonary fibrosis, hyperpigmentation, secondary malignancies, nonspecific dermatitis.

3. Nitrosoureas

    Bind through an alkyl or a carbamoyl moiety; are highly lipophilic and cross the blood-brain barrier; bone marrow depression is delayed (may be prolonged).

4. Busulfan

    Oral; bone marrow depression is selective for granulocytes; used to treat chronic granulocytic leukemia.

C. ANTIMETABOLITES

    Act primarily by inhibiting DNA synthesis; inhibit cells in S-phase (except 5-FU which has no clear-cut phase specificity); may be incorporated into DNA and RNA; major toxicity is bone marrow depression. The purine and pyrimidine analogs require "lethal synthesis" for activity.

1. Methotrexate: Folic acid analogue, competitively inhibits dihydrofolate reductase; oral, i.v., intrathecal; 50% bound to plasma proteins (displaced by salicylates, sulfonamides, etc.); excreted unchanged in urine (caution in patients with renal damage); is sometimes used in very high doses with leucovorin rescue; oral and GI ulceration, bone marrow depression are dose-limiting toxicities; hepatic and renal damage, pulmonary syndrome, alopecia, cutaneous reactions, infertility; drug of choice for gestational choriocarcinoma; used in the treatment of psoriasis.

2. Mercaptopurine: Purine analogue, major mechanisms of action are psuedofeedback inhibition of the first step in purine biosynthesis (inhibits phosphoribosyl phosphate amidotransferase) and inhibition of purine interconversions; oral; metabolism to inactive products is inhibited by allopurinol; immunosuppressive; bone marrow depression is major toxicity; liver damage, oral and GI ulcers.

3. Thioguanine: Like mercaptopurine EXCEPT allopurinol does not interfere with its inactivation.

4. Fluorouracil: Pyrimidine analogue, cytotoxicity is associated with inhibition of thymidylate synthesis and incorporation into RNA; NO cycle phase specificity; i.v.; rapidly metabolized in liver, enters CSF; oral and GI ulcers, bone marrow depression are dose-limiting; neurological defects (cerebellar); pigmentation, alopecia, dermatitis.

5. <u>Cytarabine</u>: A pyrimidine analogue (cytosine arabinoside); incorporation into DNA inhibits DNA synthesis; i.v., is rapidly deaminated in liver, plasma, and other tissues; bone marrow depression is major toxicity; oral ulceration, hepatic damage.

D. ANTIBIOTICS

So called because they are isolated from different species of <u>Streptomyces</u>; act by binding to DNA (noncovalently, by intercalation) and altering its function; cycle phase nonspecific; bone marrow depression is the major toxicity, EXCEPT for bleomycin.

1. <u>Dactinomycin (Actinomycin D)</u>

Intercalates between G-C pairs in double-stranded DNA, inhibits DNA-directed RNA synthesis; equally cytotoxic to proliferating and stationary cells; i.v., local inflammation and phlebitis; bone marrow toxicity is dose limiting; oral and GI ulceration, alopecia, acneform skin lesions.

2. <u>Doxorubicin (Adriamycin)</u>

Possible mechanisms of action include: inhibition of DNA and RNA synthesis due to intercalation, DNA fragmentation from reactive oxygen species, inhibition of DNA topoisomerase II, and interaction with cell membranes; broad spectrum of antitumor activity; i.v., extravasation with severe local reaction and necrosis, extensively metabolized in liver and excreted into bile (decrease dose in presence of hepatic dysfunction); drug and metabolites color urine red. Bone marrow depression is dose-limiting; <u>cardiotoxicity</u> (refractory congestive heart failure) is due to avid uptake by and oxidative damage to heart muscle, is delayed many months, is related to total dose administered, may be irreversible. Other toxicities, alopecia, stomatitis, hyperpigmentation.

3. <u>Plicamycin (Mithramycin)</u>

Inhibits RNA synthesis; i.v.; is highly toxic; produces hemorrhagic diathesis and bone marrow depression. Used in lower doses to treat hypercalcemia.

4. <u>Bleomycin</u>

A mixture of complex glycopeptides; causes strand scission of DNA by producing reactive oxygen species; is unusual in that it produces very little bone marrow depression; i.v.; is enzymatically inactivated in a number of tissues, toxicity occurs in tissues with low inactivating activity, 50% is excreted unchanged in urine; pulmonary toxicity (pneumonitis and fibrosis) is dose-limiting, most common toxic effects involve skin and mucous membranes; other toxicities, alopecia, chills and fever; fulminating reaction (anaphalactoid) in patients with lymphomas.

E. ANTIMITOTICS

The vinca alkaloids, vincristine and vinblastine are structurally similar but have different activities and toxicities, and no cross-resistance. Bind to tubulin, inhibit mitotic spindles, arrest cells in M phase; given i.v. (extravasation and local reaction); excreted into bile (caution in patients with obstructive jaundice).

1. <u>Vincristine</u>: Neurological toxicities are dose-limiting, suppression of achilles tendon reflex and paresthesias appear first, followed by other peripheral neuropathies, neuritic pain, constipation, disorders of cranial nerve function; alopecia; mild bone marrow depression (vincristine is considered to be marrow sparing compared to other agents).

2. <u>Vinblastine</u>: Bone marrow depression is dose-limiting; other toxicities, alopecia, stomatitis, peripheral neuropathy (neuropathy is less frequent and less serious than with vincristine).

F. STEROID HORMONES AND ANTIHORMONES

Hormonal therapy in the form of ablation, treatment with hormones in pharmacologic doses or antihormone treatment is effective for some cancers; in breast cancer, demonstration of the presence of estrogen receptors identifies those tumors most likely to respond to hormonal therapy. The use of hormones is largely empirical; they may inhibit tumor growth directly or oppose the effects of endogenous hormones. Toxicities are due to hormonal effects rather than effects on proliferating tissues.

1. <u>Corticosteroids (prednisone, prednisolone)</u>: Lympholytic; used in combination with other agents to treat lymphomatous cancers; are not myelosuppressive; mental aberrations, gastric ulcers, glucose intolerance, osteoporosis, hypertension, cataract formation, sodium and water retention, immunosuppressive.

2. <u>Estrogens (diethylstilbesterol, ethinyl estradiol)</u>: used in breast cancer, prostate cancer; nausea and vomiting, fluid retention, hypercalcemia, femininization, increased frequency of vascular accidents.

3. <u>Antiestrogen (tamoxifen)</u>: Antiestrogen, used in breast cancer; nausea and vomiting, hot flashes, hypercalcemia.

4. <u>Leuprolide</u>: A GnRH agonist, used in prostate cancer; hot flashes.

G. MISCELLANEOUS

1. <u>Cisplatin</u>: Cis-diaminedichloroplatinum (II); mechanism of action is not completely resolved, probably acts by forming DNA cross-links; i.v., 90% bound to plasma proteins, concentrates in liver, kidney, intestines and ovary, excreted in urine; renal damage is dose-limiting (is decreased by prehydration and concomittant mannitol diuresis); other toxicities: moderate bone marrow depression, ototoxicity.

2. <u>Procarbazine</u>: Mechanism of action unknown; not cross resistant with other anticancer drugs; oral; bone marrow depression is dose-limiting; CNS depression (may act synergistically with phenothiazines, barbiturates).

3. <u>Etoposide (VP-16-213)</u>: Inhibits DNA topoisomerase II; leukopenia is dose-limiting, other toxicities include alopecia, stomatitis, nausea and vomiting, neuropathy.

H. IMMUNOSUPPRESSIVE AGENTS

1. <u>Cyclosporine</u>: Cyclic undecapeptide; prevents T lymphocyte activation at
    an early stage; oral or i.v., 90% bound, fully metabolized; prophylaxis of
    organ rejection; major toxicity is renal, others: hepatoxicity, increased
    susceptibility to infection and development of lymphomas.

2. <u>Azathioprine</u>: Similar to mercaptopurine but greater immunosuppressive
    activity.

3. <u>Anticancer drugs</u>: Cyclophosphamide, methotrexate, others.

4. <u>Glucocorticoids</u>: Prednisone, others.

I. STUDY AIDE

    The table below summarizes the major mechanism of action and dose-limiting
toxicity for each group of cancer chemotherapeutic drugs. Fill in one or two
distinguishing characteristic(s) for each individual agent. Some examples are
given.

DRUG	ACTION	TOXICITY
<u>Alkylating agents</u>:	Bind covalently to DNA; inhibit DNA synthesis; cycle phase nonspecific	Bone marrow depression
Busulfan		
Cyclophosphamide	Reqs. activ. by cyt P-450; alopecia, hemorrhagic cystitis	
Mechlorethamine		
Nitrosoureas		
<u>Antimetabolites</u>:	Inhibit DNA synthesis; S-phase specific (except FU); require lethal synth. (except MTX)	Bone marrow depression, oral and GI ulceration, (hepatotoxicity)
Cytarabine		
Fluorouracil		
Mercaptopurine	Reduce dose with allopurinol	
Methotrexate		
Thioguanine		

DRUG	ACTION	TOXICITY
Antibiotics:	Bind to DNA by intercalation, inhibit DNA or RNA synth.; cycle phase nonspecific	Bone marrow depression (except BLEO)
Bleomycin	Pulmonary toxicity, cutaneous reactions	
Dactinomycin		
Doxorubicin (Adriamycin)		
Plicamycin	Used for hypercalcemia	hemorrhagic diathesis
Antimitotics:	Bind to tubulin, inhibit mitotic spindles, M-phase specific	Bone marrow depression, neurotoxicity
Vinblastine		
Vincristine		
Hormones:	Alter hormonal environm., mainly palliative	Fluid retention, hypercalcemia
Estrogens		
Corticosteroids		
Antiestrogens		
Leuprolide		
Miscellaneous:		
Procarbazine:	Unknown	Bone marrow depression
Cisplatin:	Crosslinks DNA	Renal damage, bone marrow depression, ototoxicity
Etoposide:	Inhibition of DNA topoisomerase	Bone marrow depression

CHEMOTHERAPY OF PARASITIC DISEASES

I. PROTOZOAN INFECTIONS

A. AMEBICIDAL DRUGS (Entamoeba histolytica)

   1. METRONIDAZOLE

       Agent of choice in all forms of amebiasis except asymptomatic
   cyst carriers; also useful for trichomoniasis and lambliasis; acts
   by inhibiting unique electron transfer steps; it has a direct
   amebicidal effect and is effective against systemic and intestinal
   forms; orally effective; produces cures; leukopenia, alcohol
   intolerance (disulfiram-like reaction), and rash.

   2. DILOXANIDE FUROATE

       The agent of choice in treating asymptomatic cyst carriers;
   yields cures; cheap; apparently lacks serious side effects in man -
   flatulence is common; ineffective against hepatic abcess unless
   combined with another drug.

   3. Alternate Drugs

      a. Paromomycin

          Poorly absorbed; mechanism unknown; in addition to
      eliminating intestinal bacteria, paromomycin directly kills
      trophozoites and can be used to treat mild intestinal disease.
      Also kills intestinal cestodes.

      b. Iodoquinol (Di-iodohydroxyquin)

          Directly amebicidal to trophozoite and cysts; used for
      intestinal amebiasis; ineffective in acute amebic dysentry;
      prominent toxicity.

      c. Emetine - dehydroemetine

          Used for acute amebic dysentery and extraintestinal forms
      in combination with chloroquine. Directly cidal to
      trophozoite; not effective on cysts. GI irritation and cardiac
      toxicity are common.

      d. Chloroquine

          Useful for hepatic amebiasis only when metronidazole
      therapy is not successful; ineffective for intestinal
      amebiasis. (See section on antimalarial drugs for additional
      comments on chloroquine).

THERAPEUTIC REGIMENS FOR AMEBIASIS

	Drug of Choice	Alternates
Asymptomatic cyst passer (intestinal cysts)	Diloxanide	Paromomycin
Mild intestinal disease (intestinal trophozoites)	Metronidazole followed by Diloxanide	Paromomycin
Severe intestinal disease	Metronidazole followed by Diloxanide	Dehydroemetine followed by Iodoquinol
Extraintestinal disease (hepatic abcess)	Metronidazole followed by Diloxanide	Dehydroemetine followed by Chloroquine and Iodoquinol

B. **GIARDIASIS (Giardia lamblia)**

1. **Quinacrine:** Is the drug of choice with metronidazole the alternative therapy. (See section on antimalarial drugs for comments on quinacrine.)

C. **LEISHMANIASIS (Leishmania braziliensis, mexicana and other species)**

1. **Stibogluconate sodium:** A pentavalent antimonial, is considered the drug of choice for the treatment of leishmaniasis.

D. **ANTIMALARIAL DRUGS (Plasmodium vivax, falciparum, ovale and malariae)**

1. **CHLOROQUINE**

Blood schizonticide, not effective on liver forms; rapidly and almost completely absorbed after oral administration; distributed to total body water; accumulated in the liver (this suggested its use for hepatic amebiasis); slowly excreted. Toxicity: dose related, ocular toxicity - retinopathy and corneal deposits which suggest a "bulls-eye"; GI distress, CNS hyperexcitability, and rashes. Methemoglobinemia and hemolytic anemia in individuals with G-6-PD deficiency (genetic).

2. **PRIMAQUINE**

Can destroy exo-erythrocytic, liver-lurking forms; metabolized to active forms by liver; rapidly absorbed after oral administration; toxicity: anorexia, nausea, vomiting, cramps. Methemoglobinemia and hemolytic anemia in individuals with G-6-PD deficiency (genetic).

3. <u>QUININE</u>

   Traditional agent now largely replaced by newer drugs; still
useful in drug-resistant strains of <u>P. falciparum</u>; orally absorbed;
toxicity: cinchonism (headache, tinnitus, diploplia); allergic
skin rashes; hypotension, myocardial depression, and renal damage;
intravascular hemolysis. Methemoglobinemia and hemolytic anemia in
individuals with G-6-PD deficiency (genetic). All quinone
antimalarials (QUINS) possess this genetically determined toxicity.

4. <u>DIHYDROFOLATE REDUCTASE INHIBITORS</u>

	t 1/2	relative potency
PYRIMETHAMINE	4 days	1X
TRIMETHOPRIM	14 hours	1/10X
CHLOROGUANIDE	4-6 hours	1/140X

   All compounds act by inhibiting dihydrofolic acid reductase.
Resistance to one usually confers resistance to all.
   Synergism is obtained when sulfonamides or sulfones are given
concurrently.
   All three drugs can cause weak inhibition of human dihydrofolic
acid reductase, which results in megaloblastic anemia. Folinic
acid will remedy the anemia without interfering with the
chemotherapy.
   All three drugs act <u>slowly</u>. Erythrocytic and exoerythrocytic
forms are inhibited.

5. <u>MEFLOQUINE</u>

   New antimalarial developed for treatment and prevention of
chloroquine resistant <u>P. falciparum</u>.

6. <u>QUINACRINE</u>

   Old antimalarial agent now used primarily for tapeworms; skin
may be stained yellow.

E. <u>PNEUMOCYSTOSIS</u> (<u>Pneumocystis carinii</u>)

1. <u>Trimethoprim</u> - <u>sulfamethoxazole</u>, given in combination, is
   considered the treatment of choice for pneumocystosis.

F. <u>TRICHOMONIASIS</u> (<u>Trichomonas vaginalis</u>)

1. <u>Metronidazole</u>: Is the drug of choice for treatment of
   trichomoniasis.

II. <u>METAZOAN INFECTIONS</u>

A. <u>NEMATODE INFECTIONS</u> (Roundworm)

	Drug of Choice	Alternate Therapy
Roundworm (<u>Ascaris lumbricoides</u>)	Mebendazole* or Pyrantal*	Piperazine
Pinworm (<u>Enterobius vermicularis</u>)	Mebendazole* or Pyrantel*	

Hookworm
   (<u>Necator americanus</u>) and
   (<u>Ancylostoma duodenale</u>)
	Mebendzole* or
	Pyrantel*	

Threadworm (<u>Strongyloides stercoralis</u>)	Thiabendazole	Mebendazole
Trichinosis (<u>Trichinella spiralis</u>)	Thiabendazole	Mebendazole
Whipworm (<u>Trichuris trichiura</u>)	Mebendazole	Pyrantel

*Given in a single oral dose; repeated 2 weeks later.

1. <u>Mebendazole</u>: Mostly unabsorbed. Inhibits glucose uptake, larval
    development. Few side effects: occasional abdominal distress and
    diarrhea. Contraindicated: pregnancy, allergy to drug.

2. <u>Pyrantel</u>: Paralyzes worm by noncompetitive depolarizing
    neuromuscular block. Mutual antagonism with piperazine. Some mild
    and transient G.I., CNS, skin, and hepatic reactions.

3. <u>Thiabendazole</u>: Rapidly absorbed; larvicidal for cutaneous larvae
    migrans. Frequent mild, transient side effects (vomiting, nausea,
    lethargy, dizziness) reduced by giving after meals. Cautions:
    Hepatic disease; higher doses diminish mental alertness.

4. <u>Piperazine</u>: Produces competitive block of ACh on worm muscle;
    worms are paralyzed and eliminated alive; well absorbed; mild
    transient G.I. effects and rash.

B. <u>CESTODE INFECTIONS</u> (Flatworm)

	Drug of Choice	Alternate Therapy

Beef tapeworm
  (<u>Taenia saginata</u>)
 	
Pork tapeworm
  (<u>Taenia solium</u>)
	Praziquantil	Niclosamide

Fish tapeworm (<u>Diphyllobothrium latum</u>)	Praziquantil	Niclosamide
Dwarf tapeworm (<u>Hymenolepiasis nana</u>)	Praziquantil	Niclosamide

1. <u>Praziquantel</u>: New broad-spectrum antihelminthic effective for a
    variety of cestode and trematode infections. Well absorbed; well
    tolerated; no major adverse effects have been reported; increases
    permeability of cell membrane to Ca^{++}, causing spastic paralysis of
    worm muscle, followed by disintegration of its tegument.

2. <u>Niclosamide</u>: Not absorbed. Inhibits oxidative phosphorylation and
    glucose uptake. Infrequent, mild G.I. upset.
    (NOTE: <u>Taenia solium</u> cysticercosis: Use antiemetics and
    post-therapy purgation).

C. <u>TREMATODE INFECTIONS</u> (Fluke)

	Drug of Choice	Alternate Therapy
<u>Schistosmiasis</u> (<u>Blood fluke</u>)	Praziquantil	---
Faciolopsis (<u>Intestinal fluke</u>)	Praziquantil	---
<u>Clonorchis</u> and <u>Fasciola hepatica</u> (<u>Liver fluke</u>)	Praziquantil	---
<u>Paragonimus</u> (<u>Lung fluke</u>)	Praziquantil	---

REVIEW QUESTIONS

ONE BEST ANSWER

1. _______ Which one of the following is the drug of choice in the treatment of amebic hepatic abscess?

    1. Emetine
    2. Metronidazole
    3. Chloroquine
    4. Iodoquinol
    5. Oxytetracycline

2. _______ All of the following are effective against *intestinal* amebiasis EXCEPT:

    1. Metronidazole
    2. Chloroquine
    3. Iodoquinol
    4. Paromomycin
    5. Diloxanide furoate

3. _______ Which one of the following is the drug of choice in acute amebic dysentery?

    1. Chloroquine
    2. Iodoquinol
    3. Dehydroemetine
    4. Metronidazole
    5. Diloxanide furoate

4. _______ Which one of the following is the drug of choice in the treatment of asymptomatic amebic cyst carriers EXCEPT:

    1. Emetine
    2. Iodoquinol
    3. Diloxanide furoate
    4. Metronidazole

5. _______ Which one of the following drugs would be most effective in producing a radical cure of a plasmodium vivax infection?

    1. Chloroquine
    2. Pyrimethamine
    3. Primaquine
    4. Quinacrine
    5. Quinidine

ONE BEST ANSWER

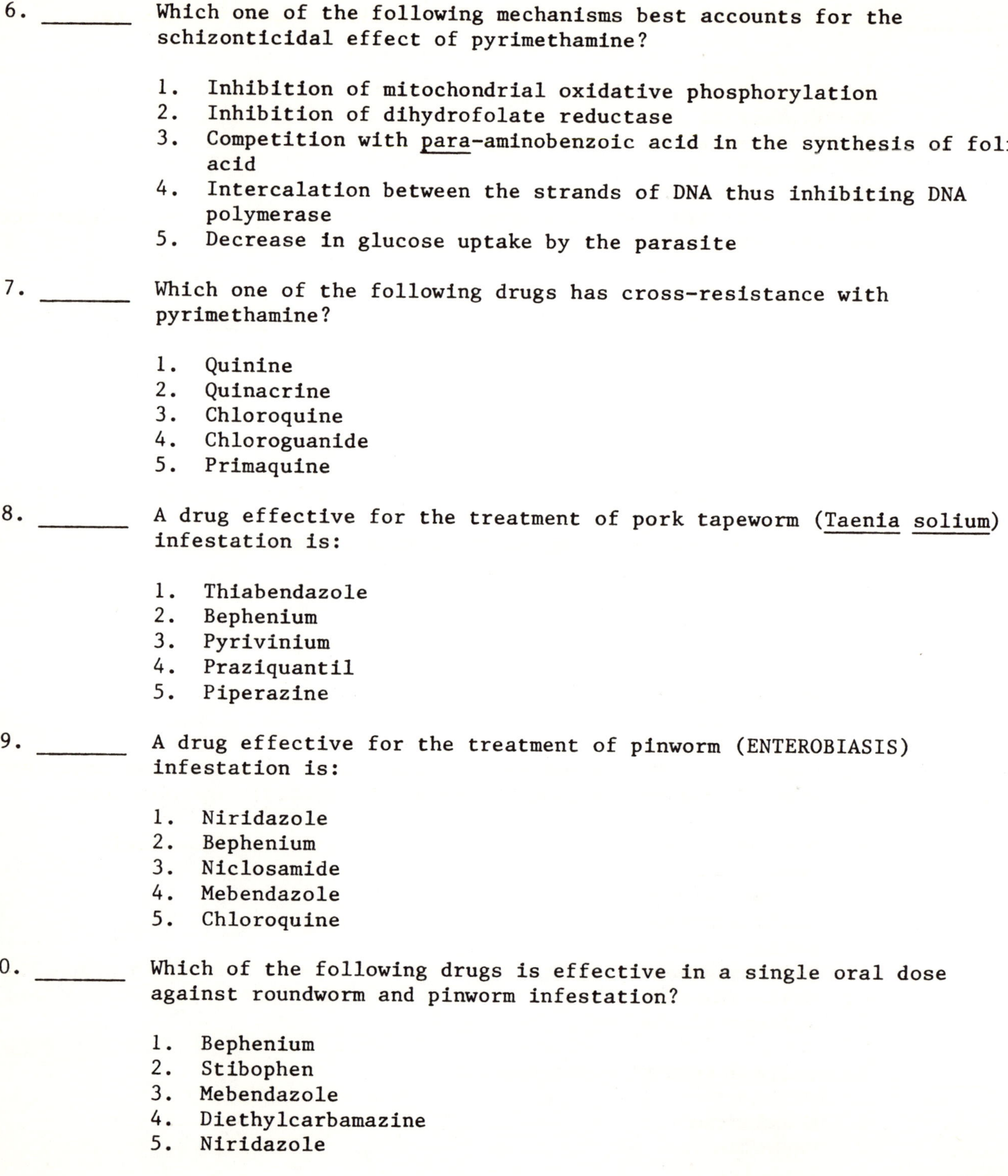

6. _______ Which one of the following mechanisms best accounts for the schizonticidal effect of pyrimethamine?

1. Inhibition of mitochondrial oxidative phosphorylation
2. Inhibition of dihydrofolate reductase
3. Competition with <u>para</u>-aminobenzoic acid in the synthesis of folic acid
4. Intercalation between the strands of DNA thus inhibiting DNA polymerase
5. Decrease in glucose uptake by the parasite

7. _______ Which one of the following drugs has cross-resistance with pyrimethamine?

1. Quinine
2. Quinacrine
3. Chloroquine
4. Chloroguanide
5. Primaquine

8. _______ A drug effective for the treatment of pork tapeworm (<u>Taenia solium</u>) infestation is:

1. Thiabendazole
2. Bephenium
3. Pyrivinium
4. Praziquantil
5. Piperazine

9. _______ A drug effective for the treatment of pinworm (ENTEROBIASIS) infestation is:

1. Niridazole
2. Bephenium
3. Niclosamide
4. Mebendazole
5. Chloroquine

10. _______ Which of the following drugs is effective in a single oral dose against roundworm and pinworm infestation?

1. Bephenium
2. Stibophen
3. Mebendazole
4. Diethylcarbamazine
5. Niridazole

<u>ONE BEST ANSWER</u>

11. ________ A drug effective in the treatment of hookworm infestations is:

    1. Praziquantil
    2. Iodoquinol
    3. Piperazine
    4. Niridazole
    5. Mebendazole

12. ________ Which one of the following drugs is resistant to acid destruction but susceptible to penicillinase destruction?

    1. Dicloxacilln
    2. Methicillin
    3. Oxacillin
    4. Penicillin G
    5. Penicillin V

13. ________ Chloramines do all of the following EXCEPT:

    1. Slowly release chlorine, which associates to hypochlorous acid
    2. Dissolve blood clots
    3. Get used for emergency sterilization of drinking water
    4. Get inactivated by protein
    5. Act better at high pH

14. ________ All of the following are true of ordinary soaps EXCEPT:

    1. Anionic agents
    2. More effective at low pH
    3. Cationic agents
    4. More effective against Gram positive than Gram negative organisms
    5. Neutralized by quarternary (tetrasubstituted) ammoniam ions.

15. ________ Which of the following drugs is most useful in ophthalmologic problems?

    1. Sulfamethoxazole
    2. Sulfacetamide
    3. Sulfadiazine
    4. Sulfasalazine
    5. Sulfamethizole

16. ________ An orally effective cephalosporin:

    1. Moxalactam
    2. Cephalothin
    3. Cephalexin
    4. Cefazolin
    5. Cefoxitin

<u>ONE BEST ANSWER</u>

17. _______ Triple sulfa mixtures take advantage of additive antibacterial
effects and non-additive:

1. Drug-resistance
2. Hypersensitization properties
3. Solubility properties
4. Binding to plasma proteins
5. Distribution to body water

18. _______ Which one of the following drugs is both orally effective and
penicillinase resistant?

1. Ampicillin
2. Methicillin
3. Oxacillin
4. Penicillin G
5. Penicillin V

19. _______ Methotrexate mostly kills cells in which phase of the cell cycle?

1. G_1
2. S
3. G_2
4. M
5. Relatively non-specific with regard to cell-cyle

20. _______ Lethal synthesis is the activation of drugs to metabolites which
produce selective toxic effects. All of the drugs below undergo
lethal synthesis EXCEPT:

1. Idoxuridine
2. Cytarabine
3. Cyclophosphamide
4. Amantadine
5. Mercaptopurine

21. _______ Vincristine arrests cells in which phase of the cell cycle:

1. G_1
2. S
3. G_2
4. M
5. Relatively non-specific with regard to cell-cycle

22. _______ Which one of the following drugs has the greatest selective toxicity
for herpes simplex virus?

1. Vidarabine
2. Idoxuridine
3. Ribavirin
4. Acyclovir
5. Amantadine

<u>ONE BEST ANSWER</u>

23. _______ A drug with selective toxicity for the granulocytic series of white blood cells is:

    1. Mercaptopurine
    2. Mechlorethamine
    3. Cyclosporin
    4. Busulfan
    5. Prednisone

24. _______ Concomitant administration of allopurinol necessitates a reduction in the dosage of:

    1. Mercaptopurine
    2. Methotrexate
    3. Thioguanine
    4. Mechlorethamine
    5. Fluorouracil

25. _______ Impairment of renal function is the major toxicity for:

    1. Tamoxifen
    2. Bleomycin
    3. Cytarabine
    4. Lomustine
    5. Cisplatin

26. _______ A "monobactam" antibiotic:

    1. Clavulanic acid
    2. Mezlocillin
    3. Imipenem
    4. Moxalactam
    5. Aztreonam

27. _______ Combinations of antibiotics are sometimes used together to achieve synergistic antibacterial effects. Which of the following combinations are synergistic because they affect a common bacterial biosynthetic pathway at two different points?

    1. Ampicillin plus gentamicin
    2. Clavulanic acid plus ticarcillin
    3. Tetracycline and penicillin G
    4. Sulfamethoxazole plus trimethoprim
    5. Methenamine plus mandelic acid

<u>ONE BEST ANSWER</u>

28. _______ A penicillin which is especially indicated for infections due to
<u>Pseudomonas aeruginosa</u>:

    1. Amoxicillin
    2. Dicloxacillin
    3. Ticarcillin
    4. Nafcillin
    5. Penicillin V

29. _______ This substance was synthesized to inhibit the renal peptidase
metabolism of the antibiotic with which it is always administered:

    1. Clavulanic acid
    2. Cilistatin
    3. Mandelic acid
    4. Amdinocillin
    5. Trimethoprim

30. _______ Its only indication is the "one shot" treatment of gonorrhea:

    1. Spectinomycin
    2. Vancomycin
    3. Amikacin
    4. Lincomycin
    5. Bacitracin

31. _______ A tetracycline which is well absorbed from the G.I. tract, even if
taken with food.

    1. Tetracycline
    2. Demeclocycline
    3. Methacycline
    4. Doxycycline
    5. Chlortetracycline

32. _______ A narrow spectrum, bacteriostatic drug, which inhibits bacterial
protein synthesis by binding at the bacterial 50S ribosomal subunit:

    1. Erythromycin
    2. Chloramphenicol
    3. Tetracycline
    4. Streptomycin
    5. Nalidixic acid

ONE BEST ANSWER

33. _______ An analog of mercaptopurine that is used as an immunosuppressant in allotransplantation procedures:

    1. Azathioprine
    2. Allopurinol
    3. Cisplatin
    4. Mechlorethamine
    5. Busulfan

34. _______ Which one of the following agents exerts part of its antiviral action by enhancing immune response?

    1. Amantadine
    2. Vidarabine
    3. Acyclovir
    4. Interferon
    5. Idoxuridine

35. _______ Which one of the following antiviral agents must be administered by small-particle aerosol?

    1. Interferon
    2. Ribavirin
    3. Vidarabine
    4. Rimantadine
    5. Acyclovir

36. _______ Which one of the following agents is used primarily for topical treatment of herpes simplex keratitis?

    1. Idoxuridine
    2. Interferon
    3. Amantadine
    4. Ribavirin
    5. Cytarabine

MULTIPLE TRUE-FALSE
Directions: For each of the statements below, <u>ONE</u> or <u>MORE</u> of the completions
given is correct.

    1 - If only 1, 2 and 3 are correct
    2 - If only 1 and 3 are correct
    3 - If only 2 and 4 are correct
    4 - If only 4 is correct
    5 - If all are correct

37. _______ Which of the following drugs exert their antitumor effects by
             inhibiting DNA synthesis?

             1. Mercaptopurine
             2. Vinblastine
             3. Cytarabine
             4. Leuprolide

38. _______ Folinic acid (Leucovorin) is used to "rescue" normal cells after
             massive doses of:

             1. Mechlorethamine
             2. Dactinomycin
             3. Fluorouracil
             4. Methotrexate

39. _______ Which of the following drugs have bone marrow depression as their
             limiting toxicity?

             1. Procarbazine
             2. Mechlorethamine
             3. Thioguanine
             4. Vinblastine

40. _______ PABA (p-aminobenzoic acid) can antagonize the antimicrobial effects
             of:

             1. Sulfadiazine
             2. Aminosalicyclic acid (PAS)
             3. Dapsone (DDS)
             4. Mafenide

41. _______ The following antimicrobial drugs act as oxidizing agents:

             1. Potassium permanganate
             2. Silver nitrate
             3. Sodium perborate
             4. Mercuric chloride

MULTIPLE TRUE-FALSE
Directions Summarized:

1 1,2,3 only	2 1,3 only	3 2,4 only	4 4 only	5 all are correct

42. _______ Mebendazole:

1. Irreversibly inhibits helminthic glucose uptake
2. Is contraindicated in pregnancy
3. Acts against all intestinal nematodes except Stronglyoides stercoralis
4. Is completely absorbed

43. _______ Chloroquine:

1. Is not absorbed
2. Can cause retinopathy (the bull's eye lesion)
3. Acts against hepatic plasmodial forms
4. Is bound to tissue and excreted slowly ($t\frac{1}{2}$ of about 7 days)

44. _______ Primaquine:

1. Is distributed to total body water
2. Has some metabolites with greater antimalarial activity than the parent compound
3. Can cause hemolytic anemia in susceptible individuals
4. Rapidly controls clinical symptoms in fulminating malaria

45. _______ The drug combination, prednisone, vincristine and daunorubicin, is effective in inducing remissions in acute lymphoblastic leukemia (ALL) because:

1. Each drug acts through a different mechanism
2. Each drug has a different toxicity
3. Each drug is effective as a single agent against ALL
4. Each drug binds covalently to DNA

46. _______ Amantadine:

1. Is not absorbed orally
2. Is not metabolized
3. Blocks the penetration of vaccinia virus into the cell
4. Can cause insomnia, slurred speech, depression, or paranoia

47. _______ The following antibiotics are usually bactericidal in their action:

1. Chloramphenicol
2. Tetracycline
3. Spectinomycin
4. Vancomycin

MULTIPLE TRUE-FALSE
Directions Summarized:

1	2	3	4	5
1,2,3 only	1,3 only	2,4 only	4 only	all are correct

48. _______ Antibiotics useful for anaerobic infections include:

   1. Clindamycin
   2. Chloramphenicol
   3. Metronidazole
   4. Gentamicin

49. _______ Broad spectrum beta-lactam antibiotics include:

   1. Amdinocillin
   2. Ceftriaxone
   3. Aztreonam
   4. Piperacillin

50. _______ Systemic toxicity largely limits their usefulness to topical applications:

   1. Bacitracin
   2. Neomycin
   3. Colistin
   4. Amphotericin B

51. _______ Orally effective antibiotics:

   1. Amoxicillin
   2. Methicillin
   3. Cefaclor
   4. Cefoxitin

52. _______ Beta-lactamase inhibitors include:

   1. Moxalactam
   2. Clavulanic acid
   3. Cilistatin
   4. Imipenem

53. _______ Narrow-spectrum antibiotics include:

   1. Erythromycin
   2. Chlortetracycline
   3. Clindamycin
   4. Chloramphenicol

<u>MULTIPLE TRUE-FALSE</u>
Directions Summarized:

1	2	3	4	5
1,2,3	1,3	2,4	4	all are
only	only	only	only	correct

54. _______ Orally effective drugs for susceptible systemic fungal infections
include:

    1. Amphotericin B
    2. Ketoconazole
    3. Griseofulvin
    4. Flucytosine

55. _______ Aminoglycosides reserved for use against bacteria which are resistant
to the other aminoglycosides include:

    1. Streptomycin
    2. Gentamicin
    3. Tobramycin
    4. Amikacin

56. _______ Recent advances which have improved the effectiveness of anticancer
drugs include:

    1. The use of intermittent high dose chemotherapy which allows the
patient's bone marrow to recover between drug courses
    2. The discovery of several new drugs which specifically kill cancer
cells without damaging host cells
    3. The use of combination chemotherapy
    4. The discovery several new drugs to which resistance never
develops

57. _______ Many of the antineoplastic agents produce:

    1. Nausea and vomiting
    2. Toxicity for tissues with a high growth fraction
    3. Immunosuppression
    4. Long-term survival regardless of the type of tumor

<u>MATCHING</u>

Choose the drug which is most likely to be effective in a case of:

1. Amphotericin B
2. Griseofulvin
3. Ethambutol
4. Vancomycin
5. Methenamine

58. _______ Blastomycosis (a systemic fungal infection)

59. _______ Tuberculosis

60. _______ Penicillin-resistant staphylococcal infection

* * * * * * * * * *

1. Iodine
2. Hexachlorophene
3. Boric acid
4. Chloramine-T
5. Methenamine

61. _______ Rapidly bactericidal

62. _______ Forms a persistent antimicrobial monolayer

63. _______ Slowly releases formaldehyde in an acid environment

* * * * * * * * * *

Match the antibiotic listed below with the toxicity most commonly attributed to it.

1. Moxalactam
2. Isoniazid
3. Chloramphenicol
4. Streptomycin

64. _______ Aplastic anemia

65. _______ Hypoprothrombinemia

66. _______ Vestibular toxicity

67. _______ Peripheral neuritis

<u>MATCHING</u>

1. Vincristine
2. Cyclophosphamide
3. Doxorubicin
4. Mercaptopurine
5. Tamoxifen

68. _______ Inhibition of purine biosynthesis; bone marrow toxicity

69. _______ Intercalation with DNA; cardiotoxicity

70. _______ Inhibition of mitotic spindles; neurotoxicity

71. _______ Alkylation of DNA; bone marrow toxicity

72. _______ Inhibition of estrogen; nausea and vomiting

* * * * * * * * * *

(Use each answer only once)

1. Mercaptopurine
2. Vinblastine
3. Doxorubicin (Adriamycin)
4. Methotrexate

73. _______ Lower dosage required in patients with impaired renal excretion

74. _______ Lower dosage required when patient is also taking allopurinol

75. _______ Lower cumulative dose in patients who have had radiotherapy to the heart

76. _______ Lower dosage required in patients with obstructive jaundice

ANSWERS

1.   2   The correct answer is metronidazole, which is preferred over the others because it is considered less toxic.

2.   2   The correct answer is chloroquine, which is ineffective against colonic infections. For this reason a drug effective against intestinal amebiasis (metronidazole) is preferred.

3.   4   The correct answer is metronidazole. Dehydroemetine does not eradicate cysts. Chloroquine is concentrated in the liver and is intestinally ineffective. Iodoquin is effective in the cyst passing patient but much less effective in acute dysentry.

4.   3   The correct answer is diloxanide, which is effective administered alone in eliminating cysts.

5.   3   The other agents do not affect exoerythrocytic forms of P. vivax.

6.   2   Pyrimethamine acts by inhibiting dihydrofolate reductase.

7.   4   Chloroguanide is metabolized to a compound resembling pyrimethamine.

8.   4   Praziquantel is the drug of choice for intestinal cestode infestations.

9.   4

10.   3

11.   5

12.   5   The correct answer is penicillin V (phenoxymethylpenicillin).

13.   2   Unlike hypochlorous acid, chloramines do not dissolve blood clots.

14.   3

15.   2   Of all the common sulfas, sulfacetamide is the strongest acid; therefore, its sodium salt is water-soluble at pH 7.4; suitable for topical administration to the eye.

16.   3

17.   3   The solubilities of different sulfonamide derivatives are independent of each other. Renal toxicity is decreased by increasing overall solubility.

18.   3

19.   2

20.   4   Amantadine is not metabolized and is excreted unchanged.

21.   4

22.   4   Acyclovir. Toxicity is much greater for the virus than for the host because the activity of acyclovir depends on its intracellular phosphorylation to acycloGMP by a virus-encoded thymidine kinase and because viral DNA polymerase is more sensitive to inhibition by acycloGTP than is mammalian DNA polymerase.

23.   4

24.   1

25.   5

26.   5

27.   4   Sulfamethoxazole and trimethoprin inhibit bacterial folic acid metabolism at two different steps. Clavulanic acid is synergistic with ticarcillin because it inhibits beta-lactamase. Mandelic acid acidifies the urine and optimizes the activity of methenamine. Ampicillin and gentamicin have different, but complimentary, mechanisms of action.

28.   3

29.   2

30.   1

31.   4

32.	1
33.	1
34.	4
35.	2
36.	1
37.	2
38.	4
39.	5
40.	1
41.	2
42.	1
43.	3
44.	1
45.	1
46.	3
47.	4
48.	1
49.	3
50.	1

Amphotericin B is quite toxic, but is indicated for systemic use because equally effective, but less toxic agents, are unavailable.

51.	2
52.	3
53.	2
54.	3
55.	4
56.	2
57.	1
58.	1
59.	3
60.	4
61.	1
62.	2
63.	5
64.	3
65.	1
66.	4
67.	2
68.	4
69.	3
70.	1
71.	2
72.	5
73.	4
74.	1
75.	3
76.	2

SECTION VIII: <u>MISCELLANEOUS DRUGS</u>

GASTROINTESTINAL DRUGS

I. LAXATIVES AND CATHARTICS

These terms describe drugs that promote defecation; a laxative promotes
excretion of a soft formed stool; a cathartic promotes a more fluid
evacuation.
A. <u>CONTACT (STIMULANT-IRRITANT) CATHARTICS</u>
Increase intestinal motor activity and stimulate water and
electrolyte accumulation in the colon.
1. <u>Castor Oil</u>: Oil from the seeds of <u>Ricinus Communis</u>; pancreatic
lipases hydrolyze the oil to the active irritant agent, ricinoleic
acid; acts on the small intestine in 1-3 hrs; should not be used
just prior to bedtime; disagreeable taste.
2. <u>Diphenylmethanes</u>: <u>Phenolphthalein</u> and <u>bisacodyl</u> act in 6-8 hrs.
given at bedtime to produce effect the following morning.
<u>Phenolphthalein</u> is a widely used proprietary cathartic in gums and
candy; if alkaline, the excreted phenophthalein will turn the urine
and feces red; allergic reactions may occur.
3. <u>Anthraquinones</u>: Active ingredient of <u>Cascara</u>, <u>senna</u> and <u>Danthron</u>
is anthraquinone or its derivatives; act on the large intestine in
6 to 8 hrs.
B. <u>BULK-FORMING LAXATIVES</u>
Naturally-occurring or synthetic polysaccharides; absorb and retain
water; fecal material becomes hydrated and soft; may also act to
reflexly stimulate peristalsis; act within 1-3 days; intestinal
obstruction reported; some drug absorption may be reduced by binding to
these agents.
1. Bran and other dietary fiber
2. Methylcellulose and sodium carboxymethylcellulose
3. Psyllium preparations
C. <u>SALINE (OSMOTIC) CATHARTICS</u>
This group includes sulfates, phosphates, tartrates and magnesium
salts; poorly and slowly absorbed from the GI tract; retain water by
osmotic effect to indirectly increase peristalsis; watery evacuation in
less than 3 hours; approximately 20% of Mg^{++} absorbed but rapidly
excreted if renal function is normal; Mg^{++} intoxication can occur if
renal function impaired.
Magnesium sulfate
Milk of Magnesia
Magnesium Citrate
Potassium or Sodium Phosphate
D. <u>EMOLLIENT LAXATIVES (FECAL SOFTENERS)</u>
No direct or reflex stimulation of peristalsis; use limited; feces
kept soft; straining is avoided.
1. <u>Surface Active Agents</u>: <u>Dioctyl sodium (or calcium) sulfosuccinate</u>
produces softening within 1-2 days; lowers surface tension to
promote water penetration into feces.

    2. <u>Mineral Oil</u>:

A mixture of liquid hydrocarbons obtained from petroleum; retards reabsorption of water; use discouraged because of adverse effects; can produce lipid pneumonia in elderly or debilitated patients; foreign-body reactions in mesenteric lymph nodes, liver, spleen and intestinal mucosa; absorption of essential fat soluble substances (vitamin A, carotene, and vitamins K and D) may be blocked.

E. VALID USES OF CATHARTICS AND LAXATIVES: Include radiological exams of GI tract; bowel surgery; proctological exam; prevention of straining at the stool by persons with a hernia or cardiovascular disease; maintenance of soft stools in anorectal disorders (such as hemorrhoids), poisoning by drugs or foods and antihelmintic therapy (saline carthartics are often used to flush the substance-or worms out of the intestinal tract).

F. CONTRAINDICATIONS: Include colic, nausea, vomiting, cramps, undiagnosed abdominal pain, and symptoms of appendicitis,

II. DIGESTANTS

Agents used in deficiency conditions to promote the digestion of food by the GI tract.

A. <u>Pepsin</u>: Proteolytic enzyme; sometimes used with HCl to treat <u>gastric achylia</u>, in people suffering from pernicious anemia or stomach cancer.

B. <u>HCl</u>: Dilute solutions of HCl for gastric hypochlorhydria or achlorhydria; encountered in pernicious anemia, stomach cancer, gastritis and in the elderly.

C. <u>Pancreatic Enzymes</u>: Available as pancreatin, a powder from hog pancreas, containing enzymes trypsin, steapsin and amylopsin. Used where there is deficient secretion of pancreatic juice, such as pancreatitis.

D. <u>Bile Salts</u>: Once widely used to replace bile acids in pathological conditions.

III. DRUG TREATMENT OF PEPTIC ULCERS

<u>HISTAMINE H_2 RECEPTOR ANTAGONISTS</u>
<u>Cimetidine</u>: Acts specifically to block the H_2 histamine receptors of parietal cells; inhibits gastric acid secretion, both basal and stimulated secretion; promotes healing of duodenal ulcer; also useful in reflux esophagitis and for Zollinger-Ellison syndrome; inhibits drug metabolizing enzymes; binds to androgen receptor-gynecomastia and impotence may occur.
<u>Ranitidine</u>: A new H_2 receptor antagonist with a longer duration of action; does not inhibit liver metabolizing enzymes, no antiandrogenic effect.

<u>GASTRIC ANTACIDS</u>

Weak bases that neutralize hydrochloric acid secreted by the stomach; used for hyperchlorhydria or peptic ulcer; may indirectly decrease pepsin activity by increasing pH of stomach to above 4; some (those with aluminum, calcium or bismuth) inhibit pepsin activity directly.
<u>NON-SYSTEMIC ANTACIDS</u>: Have a cationic group that can form insoluble basic compounds that are not absorbed and become excreted to avoid production of alkalosis.

A. CALCIUM SALTS:
1. <u>Calcium Carbonate</u>: Rapid onset; prolonged duration; inexpensive; high neutralizing capacity; unpleasant chalky taste; precipitates in intestinal tract to cause <u>constipation</u>. Hypercalcemia has occurred during chronic usage when large amounts of milk and dairy products are ingested; can lead to CO_2 formation to produce belching.
B. MAGNESIUM SALTS
1. <u>Magnesium Hydroxide</u>: (Milk of Magnesia) An antacid as well as a laxative; insoluble; laxative effect lessened by use with $CaCO_3$ or $Al(OH)_3$, which tend to produce constipation; some absorption and retention of magnesium could produce neurological or cardiovascular toxicity; magnesium poisoning more likely if impairment of renal function.
2. <u>Magnesium Trisilicate</u>: Reacts with acid to form Si_3O_2; has gelatinous form; thought to adhere to the ulcer and form a protective coat (demulcent effect); slow onset; diarrhea may be produced.
3. <u>Magaldrate</u>: A complex hydroxymagnesium aluminate; reacts with acid in several stages; $Al(OH)_3$ formed, which reacts at slower rate; prolonged antacid effect.
C. ALUMINUM SALTS
1. <u>Aluminum Hydroxide</u>: Reacts with HCl in stomach to form aluminum chloride; reaction is slow; remains in stomach for long periods; may inhibit action of pepsin and stimulate stomach mucus secretion; aluminum compounds produce constipation; decrease absorption of the tetracyclines; may cause osteomalacia.
2. <u>Basic Aluminum Carbonate</u>: Similar to $Al(OH)_3$; recommended for phosphatic nephrolithiasis; binds more phosphate than other aluminum-containing antacids.
3. <u>Aluminum Phosphate</u>: Used to avoid interference with phosphate absorption.

<u>SYSTEMIC ANTACIDS</u>: Have a cationic group that is not capable of forming insoluble basic compounds; such agents may produce metabolic alkalosis.

<u>SODIUM BICARBONATE</u>: Highly soluble; rapidly neutralizes acid; much CO_2 produced and episodes of burping occur; severe distention of stomach produced by CO_2 may be dangerous if a gastric ulcer is present that could perforate; Na^+ contraindicated in edema or in congestive heart failure.

<u>SUCRALFATE</u>: A new drug thought to accelerate healing of duodenal ulcers by forming a protective barrier over ulcer base; forms an ulcer-adherent complex with proteinaceous exudate at the ulcer site; not absorbed; does not inhibit acid secretion or neutralize acid; thought to protect ulcer from pepsin; minimal adverse reactions, constipation; may bind digoxin or tetracyclines.

IV. ANTI-DIARRHEA AGENTS

    A. ADSORBENTS

Supposedly inert powders have been employed for the treatment of diarrhea and dysentery. <u>Bismuth Subcarbonate</u>: Heavy, white powder; given in aqueous suspension. <u>Kaolin</u>: Hydrated aluminum silicate; often given in a mixture with pectin. <u>Pectin</u>: A purified carbohydrate from acid extracts of apples or the rinds of citrus fruits.

    B. BELLADONNA ALKALOIDS

Reduce tone and motility of GI tract; comon side effects, dryness of the mouth, photophobia, blurred vision and tachycardia.

    C. NARCOTICS

These agents decrease the propulsive contractions and diminish peristalsis of the intestinal tract. The intestinal contents are delayed in their passage through the tract, allowing time for the feces to become desiccated, which acts to further retard passage of the fecal material through the colon.

    1. <u>Opium Alkaloids</u>: Most effective agents for controlling severe diarrhea or dysentery; chronic therapy leads to risk of psychological and physical dependence; paregoric (camphorated tincture of opium).

    2. <u>Diphenoxylate</u>: A congener of meperidine; high or chronic doses lead to euphoria and physical dependence; often given in combination with atropine.

    3. <u>Loperamide</u>: A new meperidine congener; as effective as diphenoxylate; little tolerance develops.

V. EMETICS

Therapeutic interventions in the treatment of poisonings may involve measures to remove unabsorbed substances and/or the prevention of absorption of remaining substance.

<u>Ipecac Syrup</u>: Derived from plant alkaloids; stimulates the chemoreceptor trigger zone (CTZ); also local irritation of the GI tract; emesis occurs within 5-20 min.; must be given within 4 hrs after ingestion of poison; contraindicated in coma, convulsions, and the ingestion of caustic (corrosive) agents; caution with petroleum hydrocarbons, may get severe aspiration pneumonitis.

<u>Apomorphine</u>: Derived by treating morphine with a strong mineral acid; stimulates the CTZ; also a dopaminergic agonist; s.c. administration usually produces emesis within 5 min.; clinical usefulness is limited because it can cause CNS and respiratory depression.

VI.   ANTI-EMETIC DRUGS

Stimulus: for emesis	Blocked by:
1. Irritation of sensory G.I. nerve endings ($CuSO_4$)	1. Vagotomy
2. Agents acting on CTZ (chemoreceptor trigger zone) in medulla (apomorphine, morphine, digitalis, i.v. $CuSO_4$)	2. Blocked competively by phenothiazines (chlorpromazine is prototype but many others are more potent)
3. Emotional or psychic vomiting	3. Blocked by sedative-hypnotics
4. Motion sickness	4. Blocked by drugs having CNS anticholinergic action a) Scopolamine and benztropine b) antihistamines with CNS anticholinergic actions diphenhydramine, cyclizine, and dimenhydrinate c) promethazine – a phenothiazine with CNS anticholinergic effects
5. Nausea and vomiting of pregnancy	5. In general, because of concerns about teratogenic effects, drugs should not be used unless absolutely necessary. If vomiting persists and conservative measures do not work, cyclizine, meclizine and promethazine may be considered
6. Nausea and vomiting of cancer chemotherapy	6. Phenothiazines (prochlorperazine), cannabinoids (nabilone), metoclopramide and combinations of these and other drugs currently being used

RESPIRATORY DRUGS

I. ASTHMA: Characterized by episodic bronchial obstruction that is clinically
manifested by wheezing, dyspnea, cough and production of mucoid sputum. In
children the presenting symptom may be only a persistent cough.

   A. <u>Acute asthmatic attack or status asthmaticus</u>:
     1. <u>Oxygen</u>: 2-5L/min.
     2. <u>Epinephrine or Terbutaline</u>: s.c. (to 3 doses every 10-15 min.)
     3. Hydration
     4. If required, <u>Metaproterenol</u> by nebulizer
     5. If required, <u>Theophylline</u> by constant infusion
     6. If required, <u>Hydrocortisone</u> by constant infusion
   B. <u>Chronic asthma management</u>: Stages from occasional mild attacks needing
symptomatic relief to very severe attacks needing oral corticosteroids.
     1. <u>Bronchodilator</u>: Mainstay of therapy – mechanism is to increase
cyclic adenosine monophosphate (cAMP) concentrations which causes
bronchodilation.
       a. <u>Sympathomimetic (adrenergic) Drugs</u>: β_2-adrenergic most
selective – most common side effect is tremor; palpitation,
tachycardia, cardiac arrhythmias can occur; caution advised
with hypertension, coronary, cerebral or peripheral vascular
disease. Commonly used drugs are: Metaproterenol,
Terbutaline, Albuterol, Isoproterenol, Ephedrine, Isoetharine.
       b. <u>Xanthines</u> – Theophylline and Aminophylline (Theophylline
ethylenediamine): Monitor serum levels, large interindividual
variability; life-threatening toxicity of seizures and cardiac
arrhythmia and cardiovascular collapse can occur at high levels
without warning signs. Nausea, cramps, insomnia, headache
common with loading doses; titrate slowly if clinically
possible; these effects common at serum concentration greater
than 20 µg/ml. Combination with β_2 adrenergic bronchodilators
can be benefical because of clinical efficacy with fewer side
effects.
       c. <u>Anticholinergic agents; Ipratropium, Atropine</u>: Inhibit cyclic
GMP; efficacy is questionable.
     2. <u>Cromolyn sodium</u>: Proposed mechanism is prevention of release of
mediators from mast cells. Prophylactic use only – "as needed" for
asthma induced by exercise or specific allergens. Alternative when
seizure threshold is a concern or excessive tremor exists. Adverse
effects are rare, gastroenteritis, dermatitis or myositis.
     3. <u>Corticosteroids</u>: Prednisone, methylprednisolone, final choice to
reverse airway obstruction. They can control thick tenacious
sputum and mucosal edema. Use alternate day therapy if possible or
short time courses. Adverse effect with chronic use.
<u>Beclomethasone dipropionate</u>: Inhaled; topical administration by
inhalation decreases systemic toxicity. Prophylactic use.

II. CHRONIC OBSTRUCTIVE AIRWAY DISEASE: Chronic bronchitis, emphysema –
devastating diseases characterized by chronic cough, expectoration,
dyspnea, progressive respiratory failure, significant irreversible airway
obstruction.
   A. Oxygen: Only therapeutic agent to alter survival.
   B. Theophylline: Benefit only if reversible airway component exists.
   C. Antibiotics: Prophylactic, of limited value; need to treat infections.

D.   Corticosteroids: Methylprednisolone may be beneficial in acute exacerbations of chronic bronchitis.

III. CYSTIC FIBROSIS: Autosomal recessive disease characterized by abnormal thick secretions, pancreatic insufficiency and increased sodium and chloride in sweat.
  A.   <u>Mucolytic Agents</u>: Used to loosen or thin secretions by decreasing the viscosity of sputum; clinical usefulness, however, is limited. Treatment is effective as simple maneuvers of posterior drainage, physical therapy, hydration, and maintaining a functional cough reflex. <u>N-Acetyl-L-Cysteine</u>: Administered as aerosol or intra-tracheally in solution; reduces viscosity of mucoid secretions; may break disulfide bonds of mucoproteins; give concurrently with bronchodilator drug for best results. <u>Pancreatic deoxyribonuclease</u>: Little effect on pure mucus; reduces viscosity of purulent secretions - may depolymerize deoxyribonucleoprotein from inflammatory cell nuclei; used when acetylcysteine is not effective; anaphylactoid reactions and bronchospasm have been reported.
  B.   Pancreatin or Pancrelipase: For pancreatic insufficiency.
  C.   Salt: With fever, excessive sweating, to prevent salt depletion.
  D.   Antibotics: For infections
  E.   Bronchodilators: If bronchospasm exist.

IV. PNEUMONIA: Pneumococcal vaccine in high risk populations: Impaired splenic function, sickle cell disease, renal failure, chronic debilitation, elderly, particularly those institutionalized. Appropriate antibiotic therapy.

 V. TUBERCULOSIS: Appropriate antibiotic therapy (Isoniazid, Ethambutal, Rifampin).

VI. ALLERGY AND HAY FEVER: Antihistamines - Chlorpheniramine; medical treatment is often for misuse of antihistamines; secondary infections, bronchitis, plugs.

VII. COUGH: Most common symptom of respiratory disease. Cough suppression (antitussive effect) may be desirable for dry, hacking non-productive cough, and also may improve healing in various forms of chest trauma.
  A.   Codeine - narcotic analgesic
  B.   Dihydrocodeine - narcotic analgesic
  C.   Dextromethorphan

VIII. COMMON COLD: No specific therapy; hydration; promote nasal drainage and relieve obstruction; antibiotics to treat secondary infection.

OXYTOCIC DRUGS AND UTERINE RELAXANTS

I. Oxytocin (See Posterior Pituitary Hormones, Endocrine Section for general information).

    A. Properties:

        1. One of 2 fractions extracted from the posterior pituitary gland; now prepared synthetically
        2. Non-pregnant human uterus and uterus early in pregnancy (1st and 2nd trimesters) is more sensitive to vasopressin than to oxytocin
        3. During 3rd trimester, sensitivity to oxytocin increases markedly and is maximal at term (vasopressin sensitivity decreases in parallel)
        4. Myoepithelial cells of mammary gland contracted - causes "milk let-down"
        5. Causes transient fall in blood pressure when injected i.v.
        6. Ineffective orally - destroyed by stomach enzymes; usually given i.v. or i.m., but is also absorbed through oral or nasal mucosa.
        7. Uterine contractions occur within seconds after i.v. injection and last about 20 minutes

    B. Clinical Uses:

        1. Relief of breast engorgement during lactation
        2. Promote milk ejection in cases of inadequacy of breast feeding
        3. Induce labor at term
        4. Control post-partum hemorrhage

    C. Adverse Reactions:

        1. Sodium and water retention
        2. Do not use in patients with uterine abnormalities

    D. Preparations

        1. Oxytocin injection
        2. Nasal spray

II. Prostaglandins

    A. Properties

        1. Stimulate pregnant and non-pregnant uterus
        2. In 1st trimester of pregnancy, PGs have low success rate in inducing abortion and cause serious side effects
        3. PGs have high success rate in inducing abortion during 2nd trimester
        4. PGE_1 and PGE_2 more potent than $PGF_{2\alpha}$ during last 2 trimesters
        5. PGE_1, E_2 or $F_{2\alpha}$ can be used to induce labor at term. However, uterine responses are quite variable. They offer no firm advantage over oxytocin.

B. Preparations

    1. Dinoprost tromethamine (Prostin $F_{2\alpha}$)
    2. Carboprost tromethamine (synthetic analog of $PGF_{2\alpha}$).
    3. Dinoprostone (PGE_2)

III. <u>Ergot alkaloids</u>

Ergot (<u>Claviceps</u> <u>purpurea</u>) is a fungus which grows on rye; extracts of ergot contain a variety of pharmacologically active substances (histamine, tyramine, etc.); ergot alkaloids <u>per se</u> are derivatives of lysergic acid; chronic ergot poisoning associated with gangrene of extremities, convulsive (CNS) effects and spontaneous abortion. Ergot alkaloids have varied actions as agonists or antagonists on tryptaminergic, dopaminergic and adrenergic receptors.

A. Ergonovine

    1. Most potent ergot compound for oxytocic effect; selective action on the uterus
    2. Can cause forceful, prolonged or sustained contraction
    3. Rapidly absorbed – orally effective; prompt onset of action
    4. Partial <u>alpha</u>-adrenergic receptor agonist
    5. Chief use – to prevent and treat postpartum hemorrhage (after delivery of the placenta); to hasten involution of the uterus

B. Methylergonovine: A semisynthetic derivative with similar properties as ergonovine

IV. <u>Uterine Relaxants</u> (Tocolytic Drugs)

A. Indications

    1. To delay or prevent premature birth
    2. To slow or temporarily stop labor in order to prepare for complicated delivery

B. β_2-Adrenergic agonists

    1. Ritodrine-approved for tocolytic use. Adverse effects include increased cardiac output, hydration, hyperglycemia, hypokalemia.

C. Magnesium sulfate

    1. Given i.v., stops contractions at Mg^{++} concentrations of 4–8 mg/ml.

D. Ethanol

    1. Given i.v. as a 10% solution. May be useful when ritodrine is contraindicated (e.g. cardiac disease).

E. Experimental drugs

    1. Prostaglandin synthesis inhibitors (Naproxen)
    2. Calcium channel blockers (Nifedipine)

TOXICOLOGY

I. Emergency Treatment of the Poisoned Patient

First check respiratory function, cardiovascular function, CNS involvement, and stabilize the patient. Then attempt to determine the identify and quantify the poison ingested, and the time of exposure.

A. Non-specific antidotes

1. Emetics:

    a. Syrup of ipecac: One ounce orally usually produces emesis within 30 min.
    b. Apomorphine: Given by injection, produces emesis in 1-3 min.

2. Activated charcoal: Adsorbs a large number of organic and inorganic compounds and prevents their absorption from the GI tract. Given orally as a suspension in doses of up to 100 grams.

3. Saline cathartics: Reduce contact time between the poison and absorption sites. Examples - magnesium or sodium sulfate, magnesium citrate.

4. Diuretics: Forced diuresis may help to eliminate compounds excreted into urine. Agents used include mannitol and furosemide.
    Urinary excretion may further be enhanced by acidification or alkalinization of the urine. Weak bases (e.g. amphetamine, phencyclidine) are excreted faster if the urine is acidified with ascorbic acid or ammonium chloride. Acidic drugs (e.g. salicylates) will be excreted faster if the urine is alkalinized with sodium bicarbonate.

B. Specific antidotes

When the identity of the toxic substances is known or strongly suspected, it may be desirable to treat with specific antidotes.

Examples of Specific Antidotes

Poison	Antidote and Comments
Belladonna Alkaloids (Atropine)	Physostigmine – anticholinesterase action
Carbon monoxide	Hyperbaric O_2 – increases both O_2 delivery to tissue and CO elimination
Coumarin Derivatives	Phytonadione (Vitamin K)
Cyanide	Sodium thiosulfate – increases cyanide metabolism Amyl nitrite, sodium nitrite – produce methemoglobin which binds cyanide
Ethylene glycol, and other glycols	Ethanol – preferentially metabolized by alcohol dehydrogenase, prevents occurrence of acidosis
Iodine	Starch – binds iodine
Methanol	Ethanol – preferentially metabolized by alcohol dehydrogenase and decreases formation of formaldehyde and formic acid from methanol
Narcotics	Naloxone – narcotic antagonist
Nitrites	Methylene blue – reduces methemoglobin to hemoglobin
Organophosphate Insecticides	Pralidoxime – cholinesterase reactivator Atropine – anticholinergic agent

II. Metal Chelating Agents

    A. Dimercaprol (British Anti-Lewisite, BAL)

        1. Effective for poisoning by mercury, arsenic and some other less common metals; not very effective for lead poisoning; given i.m.

        2. Protects essential enzymes by forming stable complex with circulating metallic poison; promotes excretion of metal in stable complex form.

        3. Adverse effects; increased blood pressure and heart rate; weakness, nausea, pain at injection site.

    B. Calcium Disodium Edetate ($CaNa_2EDTA$)

        1. Especially effective in lead poisoning; given by i.v. drip; may be useful to chelate other less common metallic poisons; not effective orally.

        2. Promotes excretion of the lead chelate.

        3. Adverse effects; renal damage, hypersensitivity reactions.

4. Disodium salt (Na$_2$EDTA) - dangerous when injected i.v. - chelates calcium; can lead to hypocalcemia and death; occasionally used in digitalis toxicity to treat arrhythmias by decreasing calcium.

C. Penicillamine

1. Chelates copper, mercury, lead; given orally.
2. Used to remove copper in hepatolenticular degeneration (Wilson's disease) - accumulation of copper in tissues.
3. Used in combination, usually after EDTA for lead poisoning.
4. Adverse effects: hypersensitivity reactions; rashes, arthralgia, nephrotic syndrome.

D. Deferoxamine

1. Chelates iron specifically; orally effective to prevent iron absorption; given i.m. or i.v. for systemic toxicity.
2. Used for acute iron toxicity, iron storage diseases.
3. Adverse effects: increased blood pressure, rashes, GI upset.

III. Heavy Metals

A. Lead

1. Acute intoxication: symptoms of abdominal pain and lead encephalopathy may be rapid in onset; severe anemia; kidney damage and death in 1-2 days; rare disorder but may occur in children and young adults exposed to a large dose of lead compounds.
2. Chronic intoxication: symptomatology falls into three main categories

   a. GI: intestinal smooth muscle stimulated; spasm and hypermotility cause intense cramping - lead colic; blood vessel constriction causes pallor and hypertension.
   b. CNS: lead encephalopathy - primarily a problem in children; early symptoms rather non-specific; decreased appetite, irritable, fatigue abdominal pain, vomiting - followed by drowiness, stupor, convulsions and coma. May lead to mental retardation in survivors; may also cause cerebral palsies.
   c. Neuromuscular: lead palsy - myopathy; fatigue, weakness; wrist drop; foot drop; involvement of extra-ocular muscles;
   d. Also see anemia due to impaired heme biosynthesis; porphyrinuria, basophilic stippling of erythrocytes; gingival lead line.
   e. Treatment: CaNa$_2$EDTA for initial treatment; penicillamine also has been used; BAL not effective.

B. Mercury

1. Acute: greatest danger is damage of GI mucosa and kidney; fluid loss leads to shock and death; treat with BAL
2. Chronic: characterized by stomatitis, excessive salivation and blue gum line; kidney (proteinuria - anuria); CNS - depression, weakness, headache, insomnia, irritability, hallucinations; treatment - BAL.

IV. Teratogenesis

    A. Most teratogenic effects of drugs occur during the first trimester of pregnancy

    B. Teratogenic effects may be species-specific, which complicates drug toxicity testing

    C. In some cases, adverse complications of a disease state (e.g. epilepsy) may pose more risk to the developing fetus than drugs used to control the symptoms.

V. Chemical Carcinogenesis

Many chemicals which are present as industrial or environmental pollutants, dietary components, combustion by-products or therapeutic agents may increase the risk of cancer development. Two main classifications of chemical carcinogens have been proposed, based on their apparent mechanisms of action.

    A. Genotoxic Carcinogens

Most chemical carcinogens are thought to initiate tumorigenesis by interacting with DNA. Chemicals may be inherently genotoxic, but many chemical carcinogens are metabolized to highly reactive metabolites which in turn damage DNA. Alternatively, chemicals could act by altering DNA replication or repair.

    B. Epigenetic Carcinogens

Epigenetic carcinogens do not appear to interact directly with DNA, but appear to augment neoplastic growth by poorly defined mechanisms. This class of carcinogens includes various hormones (e.g. estrogen, diethylstilbesterol), immunosuppressive drugs (e.g. azathioprine), solid-state carcinogens (e.g. asbestos), and promoting agents (agents which increase tumor development when given after a genotoxic chemical).

ANTI-MIGRAINE DRUGS

I. Agents Useful for Acute Migraine Attacks

    A. Ergotamine:

        1. An ergot alkaloid that causes intense vasoconstriction by a direct
            action on vascular smooth muscle; can cause endothelial damage
        2. Not used as oxytocic because it tends to cause uterine spasm
        3. Poor oral absorption; after injection, onset of action delayed;
            prolonged action (12-24 hours); also effective sublingually
        4. Caffeine enhances both the absorption and the peripheral action of
            ergotamine
        5. Chief use - migraine headache (thought to decrease pulsation of
            cranial arteries)
        6. Limitations on the total dose of ergotamine that can be taken per
            attack and per week in order to prevent ergot poisoning

II. Agents Useful for Prophylaxis of Migraine

    A. Methysergide

        1. An ergot alkaloid derivative, not useful for acute migrane

    B. Propranolol

    C. Amitriptyline   Mechanism of anti-migraine
                                                         action is unknown
    D. Calcium channel blockes

    E. Clonidine

WATER-SOLUBLE VITAMINS

Vitamin	Deficiency	Physiologic Function	Therapeutic Use	Toxicity
Thiamine (B_1)	Beriberi, neurological (dry) or cardiovascular (wet)	Thiamine pyrophosphate, cofactor for decarboxylases and transketolases; modulator of neuro-muscular transmission	Thiamine deficiency	None recognized
Riboflavin (B_2)	Stomatitis, glossitis, cheilosis, dermatitis, anemia, neuropathy	FMN and FAD, coenzymes for a number of respiratory flavo-proteins	Riboflavin deficiency	None recognized
Nicotinic Acid (Niacin)	Pellagra, "three Ds"- dermatitis, diarrhea, dementia	NAD(P), coenzymes for a number of oxidation-reduction reactions	Pellagra hypercholesterolemia	Flushing, pruritis, GI distress, hepatotox-icity, ulcer
Pyridoxine (B_6)	Skin lesions, peripheral neuritis	Pyridoxal phosphate, coenzyme for metabolic transformations of amino acids, important for tryptophan metabolism. Interacts with isoniazid, cycloserine, hydralazine and levodopa.	Vitamin B complex deficiency; to prevent peripheral neuropathy from isoniazed or hydralazine; seizure disorder in infants	Sensory neuropathy, dependency, interference with levodopa effectiveness
Pantothenic Acid	Nueromuscular degeneration adrenocortical insufficiency	Coenzyme A, cofactor for acetyl transfer reactions	Multivitamin therapy	None recognized
Folic Acid	Megaloblastic anemia	Tetrahydrofolic acid, cofactor in 1-carbon transfer reactions.	Folic acid deficiency	None recognized

WATER-SOLUBLE VITAMINS

Vitamin	Deficiency	Physiologic Function	Therapeutic Use	Toxicity
Cyanocobalamin (B_{12})	Megaloblastic anemia, Neurological symptoms	Methylcobalamin, 5-deoxyadenosylcobalamin, cofactors for metabolic pathways involving folate and for conversion of methylmalonyl CoA to succinyl CoA	Prevention and treatment of B_{12} deficiency	None recognized
Ascorbic Acid (Vitamin C)	Scurvy (Hemorrhages, loose teeth, gingivitis and anemia)	Ascorbic acid, biochemical reactions involving oxidations, collagen synthesis, steroid synthesis, microsomal drug metabolism, neurotransmitter synthesis	Ascorbic acid deficiency, idiopathic methemoglobinemia	Kidney stones, rebound scurvy, interference with anti-coagulant therapy

FAT-SOLUBLE VITAMINS

Vitamin	Deficiency	Physiologic Function	Therapeutic Use	Toxicity
Vitamin A	Skin lesions, night blindness, keratomalacia, abnormalities in respiratory GU and GI epithelium, faulty bone development	Retinal, retinol, retenoic acid; affect reproductive processes, differentiation, vision	Vitamin A deficiency, dermatologic diseases, acne	Dry, pruritic skin, desquamation, bone pain, anorexia, irritability, fatigue, hepatosplenomegaly, increased intracranial pressure, edema, congenital abnormalities
Vitamin D	Rickets, osteomalacia; decreased bone density, bone deformities	Calcitriol or $1,25-(OH)_2D_3$, positive regulator in calcium homeostasis	Nutritional rickets, metabolic rickets and osteomalacia, hypoparathyroidism, Fanconi syndrome	Hypercalcemia (weakness, fatigue, nausea, vomiting, diarrhea, soft tissue calcification); growth arrest; toxicity to fetus
Vitamin K	Increased tendency to bleed	Phytonadione, menaquinones; promote the hepatic biosynthesis of factors II, IV, IX and X	Hypoprothrombinemia from inadequate intake, absorption or utilization; drug-induced hypoprothrombinemia	Hemolytic anemia, hyperbilirubinemia and kernicterus in newborn; red cell hemolysis in G-6-P-D deficient people
Vitamin E	Manifestation in experimental animals include effects on nervous, reproductive, muscular, cardiovascular and hematopoetic systems	Alpha-tocopherol; antioxidant, protects vitamin A, prevents oxidation of essential cellular components	Prophylaxis for retrolental fibroplasia in infants; vitamin E deficiency due to malabsorption	Nausea, muscular weakness, fatigue, headache, blurred vision, GI upset, creatinuria

<u>REVIEW QUESTIONS</u>

<u>ONE BEST ANSWER</u>

1. _______ Which one of the following cathartics or laxatives would not be taken just before going to bed:

    1. Cascara
    2. Danthron
    3. Methylcellulose
    4. Phenolphthalein
    5. Castor oil

2. _______ With which of the following cathartics or laxatives should generous amounts of water be taken to avoid producing any esophageal obstruction:

    1. Castor oil
    2. Danthron
    3. Milk of magnesia
    4. Methyl or carboxymethylcellulose
    5. Phenolphthalein

3. _______ The use of which of the following cathartics or laxatives is discouraged because of potentially toxic hazards, such as pneumonia in the elderly, production of foreign-body reactions, and retardation of absorption of fat-soluble vitamins:

    1. Mineral oil
    2. Danthron
    3. Phenolphthalein
    4. Epson salts
    5. Milk of magnesia

4. _______ All of the following statements about antacids are true EXCEPT:

    1. They are used for treatment of peptic ulcer
    2. They are used for treatment of hyperchlorhydria
    3. They are weak bases
    4. They decrease pepsin activity by decreasing the stomach pH to 1
    5. Those with Al or Ca content also have a direct effect on pepsin to inhibit activity

5. _______ All of the following are side effects of the belladona alkaloids, when used for treatment of dysentery and severe diarrhea EXCEPT:

    1. Dryness of the mouth
    2. Reduced tone of the GI tract
    3. Photophobia
    4. Blurred vision
    5. Tachycardia

<u>ONE BEST ANSWER</u>

6. _______ Which of the following substances is thought to be the most effective
agent for treatment of severe diarrhea or dysentery:

1. Opium
2. Kaolin
3. Pectin
4. Bismuth subcarbonate
5. Gamma globulin

7. _______ β_2 Adrenergic agonists and theophylline are considered effective in
treating asthma because:

1. β_2 Agonists inhibit the metabolism of cyclic AMP and theophylline
stimulates cyclic AMP production
2. β_2 Agonists inhibit the metabolism of cyclic GMP and theophylline
stimulates cyclic GMP production
3. β_2 Agonists stimulate the production of cyclic AMP and
theophylline inhibit cyclic AMP metabolism
4. β_2 Agonists stimulate cyclic-GMP production and theophylline
stimulates cyclic AMP production

8. _______ The drug of first choice in the emergency treatment of anaphylactic
shock is:

1. Epinephrine
2. Norepinephrine
3. Cortisone
4. Diphenhydramine
5. Atropine

9. _______ All of the following constrict bronchiolar smooth muscle EXCEPT:

1. Serotoin
2. Histamine
3. Acetylcholine
4. Bradykinin
5. Theophylline

10. _______ Which of the following would be most useful in the induction of
labor:

1. Oxytocin
2. Vasopressin
3. Progesterone
4. Ergotamine
5. Estrogen

<u>ONE BEST ANSWER</u>

11. _______ All of the following are associated with lead poisoning EXCEPT:

    1. Porphyrinuria
    2. Extensor paralysis
    3. Abdominal cramps
    4. Encephalopathy
    5. Hypertensive crisis

12. _______ The reason that the effective measured therapeutic concentration of theophylline is lower in the infant than the adult is:

    1. Decreased absorption
    2. Slower metabolism
    3. Decreased protein binding
    4. Increased receptor sensitivity
    5. Increased receptor numbers

13. _______ Blockade of vestibular vomiting mechanisms is most likely associated with which <u>ONE</u> of the following?

    1. Anticholinergic and antiadrenergic action
    2. Antiadrenergic and antihistaminic action
    3. Antihistaminic and antiserotonin action
    4. Anticholinergic and antihistaminic action
    5. Anticholinergic and antiserotonin action

14. _______ Dimercaprol (BAL) protects against the toxic actions of certain metals because it:

    1. Combines with the blood-forming elements
    2. Combines with sulfhydryl groups in proteins, displacing the metal
    3. Forms a stable complex with the metal
    4. Increases the excretion of the metal by a direct action on the kidney
    5. Supplies sulfhydryl groups to replace those inactivated by the metal

15. _______ The chelating agent which is most effective in removing copper from patients with hepatolenticular degeneration (Wilson's disease) is:

    1. Cysteine
    2. Dimercaprol
    3. Penicillamine
    4. Calcium disodium EDTA
    5. Disodium EDTA

<u>ONE BEST ANSWER</u>

16. _______ All of the following would be of benefit in the prevention of emesis due to motion sickness <u>EXCEPT</u>:

1. Diphenhydramine
2. Scopolamine
3. Meclizine
4. Chlorpromazine
5. Cyclizine

17. _______ Morphine can induce vomiting in the recumbent patient by stimulating directly the:

1. Semicircular canals
2. Stomach mucosa
3. Nucleus of the tenth cranial nerve
4. The vomiting center
5. The chemoreceptor trigger zone in the medulla

18. _______ Teratogenic effects of drugs:

1. Are easily predicted from animal studies
2. Result in an absolute contraindication of their use during any stage of pregnancy
3. Are most likely to occur during the first trimester
4. Are most likely to occur in the second trimester
5. Are most likely to occur during the third trimester

19. _______ In chemical carcinogenesis, a "promoting" agent is a chemical which:

1. Promotes the metabolism of an inert chemical into a reactive metabolite
2. Promotes tumor development when administered after a genotoxic chemical
3. Promotes tumor development when administered prior to a genotoxic chemical
4. Is defined as an immunosuppressive agent
5. Stimulates growth of endometrial carcinoma by stimulating estrogen release

20. _______ Useful in the prophylaxis of migraine headache:

1. Ergonovine
2. Ergotamine
3. Methylergonovine
4. Methysergide
5. Dinoprostone

<u>ONE BEST ANSWER</u>

21. _______   Both the absorption and peripheral actions of ergotamine are enhanced
               by:

               1. Caffeine
               2. Propranolol
               3. Amitriptyline
               4. Ethanol
               5. Aluminum hydroxide gel

<u>MULTIPLE TRUE-FALSE</u>
Directions: For each of the statements below, <u>ONE</u> or <u>MORE</u> of the completions
given is correct.

               1 - If only 1, 2 and 3 are correct
               2 - If only 1 and 3 are correct
               3 - If only 2 and 4 are correct
               4 - If only 4 is correct
               5 - If all are correct

22. _______   Individualization of theophylline dosage is required because of:

               1. Marked interindividual variation in the oral dose-response
                   relationship
               2. Narrow interindividual variation in the serum theophylline
                   concentration to bronchodilation relationship
               3. Well-documented therapeutic range (10-20 µg/ml serum
                   theophylline)
               4. Potentially serious toxicity (cardiac arrhythmias, seizures) can
                   occur without progressing through mild, readily observed,
                   symptoms of mild toxicity

23. _______   Which of the following agents induce emesis by a direct action on the
               medullary chemoreceptor trigger zone (CTZ)?

               1. Apomorphine
               2. Hydroxyzine
               3. Digitalis
               4. Chlorpromazine

24. _______   Ergonovine:

               1. Is orally effective
               2. Can cause vasoconstriction and endothelial damage
               3. Can be used to control post partum hemorrhage
               4. Promotes milk ejection in some cases of breast feeding inadequacy

<u>MULTIPLE TRUE-FALSE</u>
<u>Directions Summarized:</u>

1	2	3	4	5
1,2,3 only	1,3 only	2,4 only	4 only	all are correct

25. _______ Drugs used in treating asthma include:

    1. Cromolyn
    2. Metaproterenol
    3. Beclomethasone dipropionate
    4. Theophylline

26. _______ A patient is brought to the emergency room shortly after an overdose of amitriptyline. Which of the following antidotal treatments might be indicated?

    1. Syrup of ipecac
    2. Physostigmine
    3. Activated charcoal
    4. Atropine

27. _______ Which of the following may be useful in the therapy of cyanide poisoning?

    1. Physostigmine
    2. Sodium thiosulfate
    3. Methylene blue infusion
    4. Amyl nitrite inhalation

<u>MATCHING</u>

    1. Dimercaprol
    2. Calcium disodium edetate
    3. Penicillamine
    4. Deferoxamine

28. _______ Used to treat iron storage diseases

29. _______ Chelation therapy of choice for lead poisoning

30. _______ Orally effective for lead chelation therapy

31. _______ Effective for arsenic poisoning

<u>MATCHING</u>

    1. Lead
    2. Mercury
    3. Both
    4. Neither

32. _______ Wrist and foot drop

33. _______ Blue gum line

34. _______ CNS toxicity

35. _______ Intense skeletal muscle contraction

36. _______ Impaired heme biosynthesis

37. _______ Fluid loss and shock due to renal toxicity

* * * * * * * * * *

    1. Carboprost tromethamine
    2. Ergonovine
    3. Oxytocin
    4. Ritodrine
    5. Ergotamine

38. _______ Orally effective drug useful in the treatment of vascular headaches

39. _______ Useful for second trimester abortions

40. _______ Uterine relaxant

41. _______ Commonly used to control postpartum bleeding

42. _______ May be useful to stimulate milk ejection in nursing mothers

* * * * * * * * * *

Match the appropriate vitamins with the symptoms of deficiency.

    1. Vitamin K
    2. Vitamin D
    3. Ascorbic acid
    4. Thiamine

43. _______ Peripheral neuritis or cardiac abnormalities

44. _______ Loosening of the teeth, gingivitis, anemia

45. _______ Ecchymosis, epistaxis, hematuria, GI bleeding

46. _______ Defective bone growth, loss of bone density

ANSWERS

1.   5   The correct answer is castor oil, its acts generally within 2 hours and would cause distress. Cascara, danthron, methylcellulose and phenolphthalein are all long acting agents, one ingesting these substances could be expected to sleep through the night.

2.   4   The correct answer would be either methyl or carboxymethylcellulose. These agents could swell as they pass through the esophagus, water helps flush them rapidly into the stomach.

3.   1

4.   4   The incorrect statement is 4. Antacids do indirectly decrease pepsin activity but by increasing the pH of the stomach to above 4. Antacids are used for treatment of hyperchlorhydria and they are weak bases, and antacids with aluminium or calcium content also have a direct inhibitory effect on pepsin activity.

5.   2   The correct answer is reduced tone of the GI tract. Reduced tone is not a frequently observed side effect but the therapeutic goal of the belladona alkaloids used for treatment of dysentery and severe diarrhea.

6.   1   The correct answer is opium. Of the agents listed opium is thought to be the most effective for treatment of severe diarrhea or dysentery. Opium acts to directly reduce the tone and motility of the GI tract. Kaolin, pectin and bismuth subcarbonate are absorpbents and have no direct action on the GI tract. They are generally less effective for severe diarrhea or dysentery.

7.   3

8.   1

9.   5

10.   1

11.   5

12.   3   Remember most clinical drug assays are total concentrations, while the free concentration is what is effective. The therapeutic range of theophylline in the adult is 10–20 $\mu g/ml$ with an average protein binding of 56% resulting in a free concentration of 4.4–8.8 $\mu g/ml$. In the infant theophylline protein binding is about 36%. The same free concentration of 4.4–8.8 $\mu g/ml$ gives total plasma (free + bound) concentration of 6.6 to 11.0 $\mu g/ml$.

13.   4

14.   3   The –SH groups of BAL interact directly with the metal.

15.   3

16.   4   Chlorpromazine is the prototypic phenothiazine that acts at the chemoreceptor trigger zone in the area postrema of the medulla. Effective drugs for motion sickness suppress vestibular end organ receptors, inhibit activation of central cholinergic pathway or central vestibular pathways.

17.   5   Morphine directly stimulates the chemoreceptor trigger zone (CTZ), while at higher doses it depresses the vomiting center. The incidence of nausea and vomiting are much higher in ambulatory compared to recumbent patients. Morphine has been shown to increase vestibular stimulation.

18.   3

19.   2

20.   4

21.   1

22.   5   These answers, with the lack of clearly defined or difficult to measure clinical endpoints are the criteria for individualization of the dose by therapeutic blood level monitoring.

23.   2   Hydroxyzine and chlorpromazine are antiemetics.

24.   2   Ergotamine constricts vascular smooth muscle and is used for migraine.

25.   5

26.   1   Tricyclic antidepressant toxicity is largely due to antimuscarinic effects which are antagonized by physostigmine. Non-specific antidotal therapy (emesis, lavage, cathartics, charcoal) are all of potential usefulness.

27.   3
28.   4
29.   2
30.   3
31.   1
32.   1
33.   2
34.   3
35.   4
36.   1
37.   3
38.   5
39.   1
40.   4
41.   2
42.   3
43.   4
44.   3
45.   1
46.   2